D1170602

Sybille Hartmann

BIOENERGETIC
MEDICINES
EAST AND WEST
Acupuncture and Homeopathy

BIOENERGETIC MEDICINES
EAST AND WEST

Acupuncture and Homeopathy

Clark A. Manning / Louis J. Vanrenen

NORTH ATLANTIC BOOKS, BERKELEY, CALIFORNIA

Bioenergetic Medicines East and West: Acupuncture and Homeopathy

Copyright © 1988 by Clark A. Manning and Louis J. Vanrenen. No portion of this book, except for brief review, may be reproduced in any form without written permission of the publisher. For information, contact North Atlantic Books.

ISBN 1-55643-018-3 (cloth)
Isbn 1-55643-017-5 (paperback)

Publishers' Addresses

North Atlantic Books
P.O. Box 12327
Berkeley, California 94701

Homeopathic Educational Services
2124 Kittredge Street
Berkeley, California 94704

Cover photograph: Prismatic Dispersions by Barbara Dorsey
Cover and book design by Paula Morrison
Typeset by Classic Typography
Printed in the United States of America by Walsworth Publishing Co.

Bioenergetic Medicines East and West: Acupuncture and Homeopathy is sponsored by the Society for the Study of Native Arts and Sciences, a nonprofit educational corporation whose goals are to develop an educational and cross-cultural perspective linking various scientific, social, and artistic fields; to nurture a holistic view of arts, sciences, humanities, and healing; and to publish and distribute literature on the relationship of mind, body, and nature.

This book is dedicated to our mothers, Bea and Zizza, without whose love and support this project would have remained a pipe dream.

Acknowledgments

The authors would like to thank the following people who have helped in the preparation of this book. Foremost, we thank Johnna Albi, who nurtured us with food and humor during the twelve-hour writing marathons, and Dana Ullman, who encouraged us when our progress faltered. Also, we're grateful to our teachers and mentors within and without the health profession who aided, directed, and inspired us over the past twenty years.

In preparation for this book we utilized many books on science, medicine, acupuncture, philosophy, and numerous other subjects. We would like to acknowledge these courageous scientists and doctors who often prevailed against the reigning dogma of their times. In Chapter Two we discuss some of these unusual individuals, both ancient and modern. We salute them and hope that their work is carried into the twenty-first century.

During the seven years we worked on this book, we were not supported by institutions or grants. Despite our clinical work, we were sometimes forced to live quite simply, "without frills," as they say. But a few generous people made our day-to-day lives more comfortable and ensured the completion of this book. Our gratitude to these friends.

Our thanks to Gustavo M. Okrassa, M.D., and Yvonne Fairweather, as well as the typists who volunteered their time: Suzanne Lane, Margot Cheel, Denise Trocher, and Johnna Albi. And our hats off to Matthew Rothenberg who performed last-minute surgery on this book, received a minimal fee, and displayed an uncanny understanding of our writing and subject matter. Thanks also to Richard Moskowitz and Ted Chapman, two homeopathic medical doctors, who provided more support than they realized.

Special thanks to Steve Borghi for volunteering his art work and graphics; to Barbara Folen for helping with indexing; and to Priscilla Wiseman for answering the phone.

Table of Contents

Foreword ix

Chapter 1: Holistic and Energy Medicine 1
Bioenergy
Bioenergy and Modern Science
New Frontiers
Energy and Matter
The Biochemical Model

Chapter 2: Bioenergetic Research Through History 27
Introduction
Biographies
Conclusions

Chapter 3: Homeopathy: A Bioenergetic Medicine 65
Health and Homeostasis
The Law of Similars
Homeopathic Drug Provings
Homeopathic Casetaking and Prescribing
Hering's Law
The Microdose Enigma
Homeopathy and Scientific Validation
New Directions: How do Homeopathic Remedies
    Interface with the Body?
Homeopathy in the Modern World

Chapter 4: Introducing Chinese Medicine 91
Chinese Thought and Language:
    A Holistic Perspective
History

Chapter 5: Ancient Medicine for a Modern World 111
  Yin and *Yang*
  Diagnosis
  The Four Examinations
  The Language of Disharmony Patterns
  The Meridians and Organ Systems
   of Chinese Medicine
  The Eight Therapeutic Principles
  The Five Phases
  The Six Energetic Layers
  Chi and Blood Patterns
  The Language of Disharmonies Continued
  Speaking the Language—
   Disharmony Patterns in Action
  Chinese Medical Therapeutics

Chapter 6: Homeopathy and Acupuncture in Practice.... 147
  Homeopathic Casetaking
  Homepathic Cases
  Oriental Casetaking
  Chinese Medical Cases

Chapter 7: Disharmony Patterns and Remedy Pictures ... 171
  Disharmony Patterns/Remedy Pictures

Chapter 8: Conclusions: New Directions 225
  Clinical Applications
  Comparisons and Contrasts
  Medicine and Beyond

Notes 247

Resources................................. 257

Bibliography 258

Index 270

1

Holistic and Energy Medicine

"By equating disease with the effect of a precise cause—microbial invader, biochemical lesion, or mental stress—the doctrine of specific etiology had appeared to negate the philosophical view of health as equilibrium and to render obsolete the traditional art of medicine. Oddly enough, however, the vague and abstract concepts symbolized by the Hippocratic doctrine of harmony are now re-entering the scientific arena."

Rene Dubos, 1959
Nobel Prize-winning microbiologist

A young man lies on a white medical table, his head resting on a pillow. Periodically he grimaces and writhes. For three weeks he has suffered from low back pain for which no relief has been found, and as a last resort he has visited an acupuncturist. An Oriental doctor, his eyes closed in concentration, lifts the patient's arm and touches the radial pulse near the wrist, then quietly moves to the other side of the table to feel the opposite pulse. The doctor is short, slender and elderly; his manner, calm and quiet; his movements, graceful. After feeling the pulse, he examines the patient's tongue and asks a few questions as if to confirm what he already knows. He beckons to a young assistant carrying an instrument tray, and from it he selects a tiny silver needle with his right hand. With his left hand he locates a point on the patient's forearm, and with a deft movement inserts the needle without a wince from the patient. After selecting a few more points, he quietly leaves the room, leaving the assistant to warm the nee-

1

dles with a moxa stick. One hour later the doctor returns to a sleeping man.

To many Westerners, the preceding scenario is intriguing. It is a different and even exotic approach to treating ill people. Whatever impression one has of this scene, whatever opinion, the fact remains that acupuncture has endured over three thousand years of this planet's history, and perhaps even more amazing, it is now gaining respect in the Western world. Acupuncture, only a segment of the opus of Chinese medicine, represents a significantly different approach to healing. Perhaps the best term for this approach is "holistic." "Holistic medicine," a common expression nowadays, is an idea much abused and little understood. This book is an exploration of the heart of holistic medicine.

In the past fifty years modern medicine has reached a peak of accomplishment. As science has become more sophisticated, the biochemical secrets of the body have been revealed in a way unprecedented in recorded history. The science of physiology, the skill of surgery, the synthesis of drugs have reached levels that would dumbfound our ancestors. One cannot argue with the benefits that medical science has bestowed on mankind, but in the transition to technological medicine something crucial has been lost. As the Chinese sage reveals, there is always another side, the *yin* and the *yang*.

This book is about a side of medicine that has been neglected in modern times, but certainly not lost. Gentler methods based on ecological ideas and the healing power of the body have been pushed aside for an aggressive style based on biochemical or surgical interventions. A more subtle approach, one that we loosely call "holistic medicine," has existed in all major cultures. Though this approach often differs in quality through various cultures and eras, there are major holistic systems that have withstood the test of time. Chinese medicine and homeopathy have not only endured, they are gaining popularity and respect in the modern age. In fact, they are the most widespread and highly-developed holistic medical systems in the world today. One is from the East, the other from the West. They originated on different continents in completely different eras. Seemingly as different as the sun and moon, Chinese medicine and homeopathy are both imbued with holistic principles. As different as they may appear, they definitely share some fundamental ideas about health and disease, a fact that supports the universality of the holistic model.

Homeopathy is a system of natural remedies that are given in microdoses according to the law of similars, "Like cures like." A substance which can cause a headache can, if properly prescribed in homeopathic dose, cure the headache. This system is not based on mysticism; it has been tested and verified. Furthermore, homeopathy is not divorced in any way from modern science. Modern homeopaths make full use of modern diagnosis and testing, when necessary, but the essence of homeopathy is based on a holistic appraisal and treatment of a person, including a detailed exam of the presenting symptom, as well as a broad overview. In philosophy and practice, homeopathy is very different from the modern "allopathic" approach which opposes and fights specific disease entities.

Homeopathy is a product of European culture, emerging from Germany at the turn of the nineteenth century when Europe was entering the Industrial Era, and the French and American Revolutions were recent memories. Homeopathic ideas, however, have existed throughout history as a part of the herbal tradition, of the mysteries of chemistry and alchemy, and of ancient Greek, Egyptian, Chinese, and Incan medicine. The law of similars can be found in the writings of Hippocrates and Paracelsus, and references to it can be found in folk medicine from around the world. However, it was the German physician, Samuel Hahnemann, who developed homeopathy into a coherent and tested system. Dr. Hahnemann—scientist, translator, and medical reformer—was a unique man, a pioneer many years ahead of his time. Ironically, we in the modern world are just beginning to catch up to him.

On the other side of the planet, we find Chinese medicine, the result of a vast collective effort involving countless generations, and the product of three thousand years of culture and civilization. Emerging from the depths of ancient China over four thousand years ago, the history of Chinese culture extends from a mysterious nomadic world of warriors and shamans to the rich and varied civilization that thrives today. China has the longest continuous civilization on this planet. Chinese medicine, like its arts and sciences, has had many centuries to flower and develop, and to create a major impact on other Oriental cultures.

Chinese medicine is depicted as a tree with eight branches: acupuncture, herbal pharmacology, diet, massage, exercise, meditation, bone setting, and physical manipulation. A highly evolved system, it includes medical texts that were written before the birth of Christ. But it is also practical and down-to-earth, reflecting a close resonance with nature, the seasons and organic life. In Oriental medicine, man takes his place within the natural world of planet and heavens as an integral part of the vast web of life. His very health and survival depend on this fact.

How can these two medical systems, arising from completely different cultures, have anything in common? Can traditional Chinese medicine, ultimately derived from shamans and folk medicine, have an impact on the modern world in this age of genetic engineering and laser beams? Why is homeopathy making a resurgence in industrial nations? And most importantly, what is the practical value of these rising holistic systems? During the course of this book, we will pursue the answers to these questions.

Bioenergy

In our research and practice, we have seen that Chinese medicine and homeopathy do indeed share theoretical and even practical links, comprising a view of health and disease that is quite different from the modern biochemical approach, though not necessarily opposed to it. Both are pragmatic systems of diagnosis and treatment based on the healing power inherent in the body, and the idea that the person is an integral whole composed of body, mind, and spirit. Although different in preparation, their pharmacopoeias are derived from the three kingdoms of nature, fully utilizing nature's vast storehouse of remedial agents. Diagnosis and treatment are remarkably developed, yet simple and practical; in every aspect, diagnosis, treatment, and prescription, a commitment to holistic integrity is maintained, and thus there is no artificial division of the essential economy of life.

Both of these philosophies of medicine view health as the well-being and vitality of the whole person, and propose that this well-being is founded on an energy that regulates and vivifies life. The Chinese call this energy *"chi,"* while the homeopaths use the term "vital force." In this book we call it "bioenergy."

The defense system of the body, the caloric energy derived from food, as well as the nervous and endocrine systems, have a crucial role in the life processes, but it is bioenergy that supersedes these individual systems. It is this force that distinguishes life from death and that gives living creatures their unique quality. Present mechanistic science claims that life is a blind force that is largely regulated by chance. But is there not some force or intelligence behind the amazing drive, complexity and sheer beauty of life? Despite all its successes and power, modern science has yet to define what life really is. Therefore, it has yet to understand health. One of the great blind spots of contemporary science is its inability to confront this enigma of bioenergy, a phenomenon that refuses to go away. How could it? It is the very stuff of life.

In Hahnemann's masterpiece, *The Organon of Medicine,* he states:

> In the state of health the spirit-like vital force (dynamis) animating the material organism reigns in supreme sovereignty.
>
> It maintains the sensations and activities of all the parts of the living organism in a harmony that obliges wonderment. The reasoning spirit who inhabits the organism can thus freely use this healthy living instrument to reach the lofty goal of human existence.[1]

In Chinese medicine we find the similar concept of *chi*. A difficult concept to define, *chi* is left untranslated because in Chinese it has many nuances and meanings, but for our general purpose we shall equate *chi* with what we call the bioenergy.[2] The great Cambridge University scholar, Joseph Needham, gives his interpretation of *chi:*

> . . . We said that *chi* is something like the life pneuma, i.e.,
> subtle spirits, tenuous matter, something resembling air, or gas,
> or vapor, but also something which could have the character of
> radiant energy like radioactivity . . . [3]

In Chinese medicine the *chi* is said to circulate through the
body in specific pathways, regulating and animating. *Chi* is the
source of all movement, not only in human life, but in the universe.
The following is a quote from an ancient Chinese text:

> The root of the way of life (*Tao*), of birth and change, is
> *chi:* the myriad things of heaven and earth all obey this law.
> This *chi* in the periphery envelops heaven and earth, *chi* in the
> interior activates them. . . . [4]

To the average Western scientist the idea of any life energy
is nonsensical. What present laws of physics and chemistry can
account for this principle? Or one could ask: what in our present
vision prevents us from understanding this phenomenon? In the
next chapter, we demonstrate how consistently this idea has been
studied throughout history, but it is only in this century that we
have approached evidence of its existence. At the end of the twentieth century, we are finding increasing proof in physics, biology,
and psychology of a unifying biological force field.

We should also mention that the bioenergy phenomenon is
one of the many natural mysteries that science has yet to resolve
fully. For example, science is currently struggling to fit such diverse
subjects as black holes and telepathy into its present model. Even
more common subjects such as electricity and nuclear energy are
not fully understood; man might utilize these forms of energy every
day, but he does not understand their precise mechanism. On a
more subjective note, how can physiology explain the mystery of
emotions like anger and love? Can love or anger be reduced to
simple biochemical reactions in the brain cells? Another interesting
question is the evolution of life forms. How can all the incredible
variations of life forms on this planet be derived from the four
basic DNA molecules? These and many other questions have yet

to be explained. Biochemical "cause-and-effect" has not yet accounted for many of these questions because of inherent limitations in the model. Perhaps a new direction into holistic perspectives, as well as biochemical analysis, will result in a more fruitful understanding of the universe.

What is this force that animates matter? Is it the biochemical reactions and electricity known to modern science? Is it some form of electromagnetism that we do not yet comprehend? Is it simply the regulating homeostatic principle of life or is it a new energy yet to be discovered? What does it mean when someone says, "My energy was low today"? One can, of course, ascribe various physiological functions to this quality, but life, to be alive, must be more than one system or function: it is the totality. Quite obviously we are discussing an elusive force that is not readily visible and palpable to the normal senses. As will be seen in the next chapter, it is not something that can be studied easily in the laboratory (much to the perplexity of our stolid physical scientists). But the fact remains that something is there, a biological force or energy that vivifies and regulates all life. This question of bioenergy is a universal enigma that has always been debated; it encompasses the realms of intuition and science, but ultimately it is an existential question in the realm of direct experience.

If the universe were static, inert, and readily measurable in all aspects, then one could analyze and define all the unknowns without any quibbling, but fortunately, the universe cannot be so simply reduced. The same is true for life. Life is a dynamic process of complex interactions that cannot be reduced without intervening with the whole. We can, for instance, dissect the body down to its most microscopic elements, but will we find the mystery of life there? Presently, science claims that we can find the mystery of life in these miniscule parts. Furthermore, our present model focuses on the part and overlooks the whole. In modern medical practice, there are now at least sixty-six medical specialities. Despite the obvious necessity of specializing, it can lead to a false perspective of the integrity of the body/mind. Each specialist will see the patient in terms of his speciality. Who is there to heal the whole person? Dr. Alex Carrel, a nobel prize-winning scientist, addresses this question: "Man as known by the specialist is far from being the concrete man, the real man. He is nothing but the schema, consisting of other schema built upon the techniques of each science."[5]

Chinese medicine and homeopathy, in their finest expressions, are founded on a holistic model of man and nature. Man is an integral part of the greater life on this planet. His internal equilibrium is a part of the general movement of life around him: the weather, the family, the society, and the general environment. The person—mind, body, and spirit—is an expression of this bioenergy which accounts for the unique quality of life. Health can be defined as a relative and dynamic state of equilibrium of this life energy. Disease is an imbalance in this equilibrium which, in time, will lead to local tissue change, pathology.

Behind these different medical systems, biochemical and holistic, we see different paradigms. For simplicity we call these paradigms "Western" and "Eastern." The Western model is linear and analytical; the Eastern, holistic and circular. The Western view sees particles or parts and wants to know the "why" of these elements, while the Eastern view sees patterns and relationships as the dominant "shape" of reality.[6] In the West our symbols are more concrete and defined, like the classical model of the atom (a model now in transition). The Eastern model creates symbols, like the *yin/yang* symbol, which are more dynamic and holistic. The Eastern model is empirical in the sense that it is based on practical observation of life in process. The living person is studied in order to understand the disease process and restore health. The Western model is more abstract, speculating first, acting, and then observing.[7] The Western biochemical model looks for disease in the malfunctioning of chemicals and tries to diagnose a specific disease entity.

We see an apparent polarity between these two models, but any artificial division promotes a limited perspective. Chinese holistic philosophy is represented by the *yin/yang* image, symbolic of the two forces of nature. *Yang* is the more active force; *yin*, the more feminine, passive force. The balance between the two is called the *tao*. The balance, never static or defined, is in dynamic equilibrium. *Yin* or *yang* cannot exist without the other; neither is "better" or "worse" than the other; hence, they should not be viewed as separate poles. They are not opposed; in fact, they exist in a dynamic interrelation from which all movement and creation result. To create a more complete view of our universe (and of medicine), we must not exclude either Western or Eastern models. Like the balance of *yin* and *yang*, the integration of both traditions is necessary for a truly universal vision.

Bioenergy and Modern Science

The concept of bioenergy has been scorned by modern science. It is, in fact, a taboo subject, and any attempt to revive it will send cold shivers down the backs of most scientists. This idea runs contrary to all the assumptions and theories of the biochemical model. In this book, however, we wish to present a modern view of bioenergy.

One of the major reasons why bioenergy is not accepted by mainstream science is because it is a holistic concept and not readily subject to the same testing criteria as conventional biochemical phenomenon. However, in light of recent advances in modern physics and other scientific disciplines, there is no reason for this automatic rejection. There is growing scientific evidence from around the world that living organisms do indeed possess a unified bioelectric force field; and with the determination of this fact, a new model of life will emerge, creating great changes in biology and medicine.

If bioenergy is more than an idea, if it is energy in the conventional sense, there must be some physical presence that can be measured and tested. In the past, one major obstacle to this goal was the lack of instrumentation subtle enough to provide proof. (Another obstacle is finding scientists bold enough to tackle this taboo area!) Almost every great scientific advancement has been based on the discovery of new instrumentation. Over the past centuries we have seen the development of the microscope, the Leyden Jar, the telescope and the cyclotron, innovations all critical to the progress of different scientific disciplines. Similarly, the evidence for bioenergy requires new methods and devices, obstacles that are now being resolved. We shall discuss some of the pioneers of bioenergy in the next chapter.

One vitally important complication in researching bioenergy is that it appears to consist of at least two energy fields. One consists of low-frequency electro-magnetic fields; the other, nonelectrical, is a mysterious subtle energy field akin to the Oriental concept of *chi*. Some researchers (Reich, Reichenbach) claim that this energy has properties that electricity does not possess, such as conduction through silk and wood. On the other hand, other researchers (Burr, Becker, Nordenstrom) have explored a unified electrical field in the body (an idea much more amenable to conventional science). Slowly, the electromagnetic fields will be recognized by the scientific community, but the other nonelectrical field will continue to be a mystery for some time.

In this book we make no pretense of unraveling all of these questions, but we do wish to explore different aspects of bioenergy, even if this task entails treading in unknown (or forbidden) territory. In our opinion, these two concepts of bioenergy are closely related, like the *yin* and *yang* of each other, and for the sake of simplicity, we will use the term "bioenergy" to connote both. We suggest that the more subtle, non-electrical field is the universal life energy (*chi, prana, pneuma*) that in living organisms has a bioelectrical manifestation.

Bioenergy is clearly a holistic phenomenon that must be studied as such, and until this perspective is seriously considered, there will be no acceptance of these new ideas. These concepts will make little sense if studied in parts from one discipline. Perhaps more credence will be given to the holistic perspective through the discoveries of modern physics. Quantum physics, at the forefront of research into matter and energy, has recently created a holistic picture of the universe. This positive direction might in turn lead to answers regarding some of the great mysteries of nature. What, for instance, is the basic unifying force in nature?

What unifies the four fundamental universal forces: nuclear, electro-magnetic, weak interacting, and gravitational? What is the relationship between these forces? No one knows the answers to these questions, but perhaps the new directions of the holistic model will yield a solution. After all, not too long ago, scientists theorized that matter and energy were separate. Einstein, Heisenberg, Bohr, and other physicists have created a new vision which is leading to a more holistic view of matter, energy, and the universe:

> "We may therefore regard matter as being constituted by regions of space in which the field is extremely intense . . . there being no place in this new kind of physics for the field and matter, for the field is the only reality."—Albert Einstein

We are entering an exciting new era for medicine, biology, and the life sciences. We believe that holistic concepts will have a greater influence in these areas. Ecology, for example, is a relatively recent discipline within biology; essentially a holistic discipline, it recognizes the importance of the matrix of relationships in nature, and creates a vision of a web of interrelationships in the natural world which man can no longer thoughtlessly ignore.

Before the reader falls under the illusion that we have a complete understanding of this life energy, let us assure you that we do not. Even though it is more than a theory in our view, bioenergy has an elusive quality, reminding us of the words of Lao Tzu, the famous Chinese philosopher: "The *tao* (way) that can be told is not the true *tao;* the name that can be named is not the true name."[8]

Even more confusing, many researchers have named this energy according to their training and perspective. As a result, the profusion of synonyms for "bioenergy" is incredible. Another complication we observed is that the concept of bioenergy encompasses two different but closely-related ideas, what Chinese philosophers call *li* and *chi. Li* is more like an etheric blueprint or idea that underlies all material things, while *chi* is the activating force or energy that animates matter.[9] *Li* and *chi*, like *yin* and *yang*, are interdependent and should not be artificially separated.

We will discuss these concepts later in the book.

Claude Bernard, the famous French physiologist of the last century, is a key figure in the history of modern medicine. He is often credited with undermining, once and for all, the Vital Energy theory which he felt—with some justification—was impeding scientific research. People at that time used life energy to account for all organic phenomena, therefore precluding any reason to look deeper into the mysteries of chemistry. Bernard meticulously studied the body from the laws of chemistry and physics and found no room for vitalism in his research. As the life processes such as respiration were explained in terms of an exchange of gases, there seemed no reason for bioenergetic justification.

Bernard's hardnosed attitude and his research certainly merit admiration, but he was attempting to bury a living corpse! The Victorian Age scientists were anxious to do away with vitalism because they were busy erecting a sterile, mechanical mode of life, and imagined that they could eradicate its last shred of mystery. Nature, it was thought, was totally within the grasp of human reason; these researchers felt that life itself was ultimately explicable in terms of the mechanical laws of chemistry and physics. Bernard was inextricably a part of this Victorian climate. He correctly assumed that the physical processes of the body are not shrouded in mystery; to a large extent they are governed by laws that can be scientifically determined. But like all great scientists, Bernard was not insensitive to the ultimate mystery of the living organism. "There is an arrangement in the living being," he wrote, "a kind of regulated activity, which must never be neglected because it is, in truth, the most striking characteristic of living beings."

New Frontiers

One of the most wonderful mysteries of life is the question of morphogenesis: how the actual forms of living things come into being. A seed of a fertilized egg has very little form, but as it develops, the embryo manifests more complexity, order and form. How this marvelous embryological development occurs is one of the central questions of biology, but after decades of trying to explain it with the biochemical model, researchers have met with little success. In the last thirty years biological science has discovered much about DNA, its structure, and how it codes the sequence of amino acids and proteins. Much has been discovered about the chemical changes in the organism during development. But this data about DNA, the smallest unit of life, does not explain why an organism—bee, rabbit, or man—takes a particular form any more than analyzing the bricks of a building can predict its overall design.[11]

Dr. Rupert Sheldrake, a research biologist and graduate of Cambridge University, postulates that something besides DNA regulates the morphogenesis of life and all the amazing variations of organic form. In his book, *A New Science of Life*, Dr. Sheldrake develops his thesis of morphogenic fields, giving evidence from embryology and other related disciplines. DNA, he explains, is simply a set of instructions; these instructions are the same in every cell, in *every* kind of living organism. All biological scientists agree that something else must act on the DNA to unlock and interpret the code, and to cause different parts of the genetic information to be expressed as each cell comes into being. Dr. Sheldrake argues persuasively for his thesis that the morphogenesis of the organism is not based on the part giving rise to the whole, but that the whole or pattern gives rise to the parts. He calls these life patterns "morphogenic fields." This morphogenic field theory is not alien to modern biology; on the contrary, it is widely respected. Paul Weiss (see Chapter Two) and other prominent biologists had previously developed ideas similar to Sheldrake's. In fact, this concept is articulated in the philosophies of Plato and Socrates. Morphogenic fields, Sheldrake explains, are patterns, not static blueprints. They determine form and structure in all living things, and like the familiar fields of magnetism and gravity, they are intangible but can be inferred from their influence on tangible things. Sheldrake emphasizes that morphogenic fields are not to be confused with bioenergy. They have no energy of their own but simply provide an overall pattern, similar to the Chinese concept of *li*.

For another point of view, we can turn to the remarkable research of Harold Burr, M.D., of Yale University, who for thirty years meticulously studied living organisms with a voltmeter. With delicate electrodes Burr could measure the electrical potential of people, plants and animals without disturbing their electro-dynamic field. He describes this pioneering effort in his book, *The Fields of Life*. Dr. Burr produced careful documentation to verify his statements. We should make it clear that he did not measure the electrical flow, or isolated electrical charges in the body, but rather the steady-state energy level of the living organism. Let us take a brief glance at his conclusions:

> The pattern of organization of any biological system is established by a complex electro-dynamic field which is in part determined by its atomic physio-chemical components and which in part determines the behavior and orientation of those components. This field is electrical in the physical sense and by its properties relates the entities of the biological system in a characteristic pattern and is itself, in part, a result of the existence of those entities. It determines and is determined by the components.
>
> More than establishing a pattern, it must maintain a pattern in the midst of a physio-chemical flux. Therefore, it must regulate and control living things. It must be the mechanism, the outcome of whose activity is wholeness, organization and continuity.[12]

From his research Dr. Burr determined that there is a unified electro-dynamic force field. Though Burr was careful not to align himself with the old-fashioned vitalists, he accomplished in his laboratory what they were not able to: he gave some scientific credence to their theory. Burr, as we point out in the next chapter, is not alone in his type of research, but he was one of the first scientists to study this force field with scientific instruments. Although Burr's research was somewhat rudimentary by today's standards, he was a bold and imaginative pioneer who had a clear vision of the important medical potential of his field. Unfortunately, the medical establishment of the 1930's was not in the least interested in Burr's discoveries, and in spite of his best efforts, his work was ignored.

We should clarify that Burr's theory of electro-dynamic force fields differs from Sheldrake's theory of morphogenic fields. Both are holistic concepts but each emphasizes a different underlying unifying pattern. Burr's emphasis is more physical, an electro-dynamic pattern, while Sheldrake's is more metaphysical, an overall blueprint with no tangible properties. Burr's concept has much in common with *chi*, while Sheldrake's resembles *li*.

Dr. Ravitz, one of Dr. Burr's esteemed colleagues, researched areas of emotional and mental health. Ravitz, a psychiatrist, used Burr's voltmeter as a means for studying human emotions; his studies of hypnotic and schizophrenic states are especially intriguing. In schizophrenia he discovered an excess of energy, an extreme imbalance, and compared it to the overcharging of a battery. In many experiments, Dr. Ravitz observed that an improvement in the patient's condition brought about a sustained voltage drop. Ravitz studied patients suffering from a variety of mental/emotional problems and concluded—as did homeopaths and Chinese physicians—that disease usually follows a drop in energy of the person. Chinese doctors call this "deficient *chi*" and consider it a precursor of many diseases. They have specific methods to build the *chi* and thus prevent the onset of sickness.

There are many other contemporary scientists who have added to this interesting body of research. From our point of view, two of the most outstanding are Bjorn Nordenstrom from Sweden and Robert Becker from the United States. Dr. Nordenstrom is an internationlly-recognized scientist with over thirty years of research experience. A specialist in radiology, Nordenstrom pioneered the needle biopsy, a diagnostic technique now used in every major hospital in the world. More important, however, have been his two decades of research into the bioelectric fields of the body, studies which culminated in the book, *Biologically Closed Circuits: Clinical, Experimental, and Theoretical Evidence for an Additional Circulatory System.* In terms of conventional medicine, this book is revolutionary, and naturally it has been ignored. Nordenstrom's major thesis is that the body contains a complex electrical system that regulates the activity of the internal organs and is the foundation of health. Sound familiar? Nordenstrom backs his thesis with two decades of meticulous scientific research. He claims that modern medical science has not adequately explored the electrical properties of the body and has yet to explain how the chemical and physical processes of the body are interrelated. Dr. Nordenstrom has also applied his theories by treating tumors with specially-devised electrical probes.

Across the Atlantic, Dr. Robert Becker has been conducting research into the bioelectric properties of the body, a lengthy study which culminated in a book, *The Body Electric*. Dr. Becker, an orthopedic surgeon, was led into this research because of his interest in the miracle of regeneration. For example, if a salamander's tail is cut off it will soon grow another, a process which modern science has yet to explain. Dr. Becker thinks that the secret lies in the unifying bioelectric properties of the body. Dr. Becker has also conducted original research on acupuncture, but, like many pioneer scientists, his career in research has been constantly thwarted by skeptical colleagues and superiors.

More evidence for bioenergy comes from Russia where a husband-and-wife team of scientists, Semyon and Valentina Kirlian, developed a new technique of photography. Their device, a result of scientific wizardry, is a high-frequency spark generator, or oscillator, generating between 75,000 and 200,000 electrical oscillations per second. Any living object, part or whole, can be photographed to reveal strikingly beautiful emanations. The device creates a high-frequency field that apparently causes living things to radiate a bioluminescence on photographic paper; this bioluminescence is said to be the radiation of the living energy, similar to the aura. The Kirlians came to this conclusion when, after several years of experimentation, they were brought two apparently identical leaves to photograph. The difference in the emanations was immediately apparent, and it was then they were told that one leaf came from a healthy plant, the other from a contaminated specimen. The Kirlians came to realize that these emanations were from a unified biological energy field.

After many years, the Kirlians' work was begrudgingly recognized by the Soviet scientific establishement, and subsequently, hundreds of eminent Soviet scientists witnessed Kirlian photography. The Kirlians were the first to develop sophisticated electro-photographic equipment, but other scientists had entertained the possibility, such as the famous Nikolai Tesla and Dr. Walter Kilner of St. Thomas Hospital in London. Predictably, there has not been a great uproar of excitement or research on this subject in America. One of the leading American researchers is Dr. Thelma Moss, formerly of the School of Medicine at the University of California in Los Angeles. She has demonstrated that the emanations from the body are not simply the result of physiological variations at the surface of the skin. On the contrary, she has found that relaxation states, produced by acupuncture or meditation, are characterized by wider and more brilliant emanations, the opposite occurring in states of tension.

While an interesting phenomenon, Kirlian photography is a controversial topic, and there are valid doubts about the ability to reproduce this phenomenon consistently. However, much of the information that has resulted from this technique is found in other areas, and the idea that the body generates a bioenergetic field is not surprising.

In this section we have presented a brief overview of bioenergetic research, a topic we will explore in more depth in the next chapter. While the past has much to offer us in bioenergetic research and writing, we believe that the future holds more, and within the next decade this field will be flooded with new information.

Energy and Matter

Quantum physics, already briefly mentioned, provides additional support for our thesis. While this research does not validate the existence of bioenergy, it certainly supports the holistic model.

In this book we cannot even touch the surface of the complex field of quantum physics; instead we refer the reader to our bibliography. It is worthwhile, however, to consider the implications of this research. Einstein was one of the first modern scientists to explore new models of the universe with his studies in relativity. He determined that matter and energy are one, thus transforming the classical Western duality, and ensuing discoveries by physicists like Neils Bohr and Werner Heisenberg decisively challenged the concept that atoms are the final building blocks of matter. Subatomic particles have been discovered that defy description as either particles or waves. These "qualities" of energy, given odd names like "leptons" and "quarks," act with indecent unpredictability, disturbing our present assumptions about matter. This subatomic world appears to be a complex web of interrelationships—one could say a "holistic pattern."

For centuries our Western model has been based on the idea that atoms are indestructible, discrete particles. This model is founded in part upon the physics of Isaac Newton, the great eighteenth-century scientist. Newton's universe is based on the duality between void and matter. Amidst this void are distinct atoms that have a mass and movement which can be measured and predicted. *En masse*, they are the discrete particles that create the solid world we see and touch. Newton's theories are based on a common-sense view of the world that we see, touch, and expect to be.[13] The solid world exists in a linear time frame and everything is governed by cause and effect. From these basic observations and calculations, Newton erected his brilliant edifice of mathematics and philosophy, the core of the present scientific world view. His mathematical laws, predicting how events will unfold in nature, gave man an awesome power to manipulate the physical world. Position, mass, and velocity are precisely defined by Newton's laws, opening up a whole new realm of physical applications which are responsible for the conveniences and comforts of the modern world.

In the past few decades, however, new facts emerging from research in quantum physics have been eroding the solid position of the Newtonian model. This does not mean that the model is incorrect; it does indicate, however, that it is incomplete. Our knowledge of the universe is expanding beyond the Newtonian boundaries, and a new picture is evolving with profound implications for the modern world. Let us quote the contemporary physicist David Bohm, a former student of Einstein:

> One is led to a new notion of the unbroken wholeness which denies the classical idea of the analyzability of the world into separately and independently existing parts. . . . Rather, we see that the inseparable quantum interconnectedness of the whole universe is the fundamental reality, and that the relatively independently behaving parts are merely particular and contingent within the whole.[14]

Physicist Fritjof Capra has eloquently discussed the interface of quantum physics and oriental cosmology in his book, *The Tao of Physics*. Other scientists have added to this pioneering effort in subsequent books. These books are not the work of harebrained dreamers but of respected scientists, and all of a sudden the Chinese concept of *yin/yang* does not sound so outlandish. The universe is indeed this vast oscillation of interconnected forces, an observation that Chinese scientists made centuries ago. In our opinion, the bioenergetic phenomenon will prove to be the web that relates all living matter. Each organism, animal, plant, or insect is unified in its form and function by this life energy, just as the universe may prove to be unified by a similar force field.

As Dr. Larry Dossey explains, these new discoveries in modern physics are not far removed from the work of healing sick people:

> Why should we attempt to view the human processes of health and disease in terms of the new physical views offered by quantum physics and relativity? In the first place, as the physicist Wheeler has observed, everything is quantized at some level: "The world at the bottom is a quantum world; and any system is ineradicably a quantum system." This suggests that eventually our concepts of how our bodies work will have to give due regard to quantum physical events and the . . . subatomic world.[15]

Whether the critics like it or not, a new image of the universe is emerging, not from some mystic fringe, but from the forefront of physical science. All sciences, including medicine, will soon have to account for these changes. Science is not absolute; it is not based on a rock foundation of unchangeable facts. Rather, it is founded on recognized conventions and variables; now these conventions—the structure of the model—are shifting. We are entering an exciting, challenging era, reminiscent of the Copernican Revolution.

The Biochemical Model

So that we may better understand bioenergetic medicine, let us examine some of the basic tenets of orthodox medicine. Molecules and changes in molecules are the central thrust of conventional medical research, while diseased tissue (pathology) is the focus of diagnosis and treatment. Biochemical evidence of this pathological tissue change is the basis for administering drugs, substances tested to alter and control the changes in molecules. Since chemical reactions are considered to be the basis of life, illness is solely regarded as a chemical malfunction. In the disease process the person is secondary to the pathology. The pathology, localized in certain areas, is the disease. Emotions, environment, and complex energetic interactions are secondary to this biochemical malfunctioning. The regenerative power of the body is given a minor role in the process of healing, as synthetic chemicals are deemed far more dependable than Mother Nature or any nebulous homeostatic mechanism.

Modern drugs are, for the most part, powerful chemicals that can control specific molecular malfunctions—this is the epitome of their strength and weakness. These drugs can efficiently eradicate proliferating bacteria in pulmonary lesions, just as they can grossly intervene in the delicate homeostasis, causing serious side effects. They can be toxic. The effectiveness of these drugs has been tested on animals in laboratories with the assumption that they will act in a similar way on humans. The weakness of this rigorous testing is that it only looks at the physical aspect of illness. The sole basis for using these drugs is the linear biochemical model where the "dis-ease" is the diseased tissue. Obviously this approach is extremely valuable in the treatment of diseases like pneumonia and syphilis, but what about difficult chronic conditions for which no clear-cut cause is found?

The biochemical model has serious limitations when dealing with disease syndromes, with functional problems, and with complex chronic diseases that do not readily respond to simple cause-and-effect. From the bioenergetic point of view, the biochemical model tends to focus on the end process of disease—the phsycial degeneration—ignoring both the mind-body connection and the existence of energy fields. It is within these fields that disturbances first manifest themselves, analogous to distortions in wave patterns; and it is here, from our experience, that the disease process can be best prevented or treated. It is in this direction that medicine is now heading, albeit slowly.

Since the discovery of bacteria by Koch and Pasteur in the last century, modern medicine has centered on this biochemical model of disease. This molecular model is founded on several concepts: linear cause and effect, dualistic perception, and the idea of specific etiology—all solidly "Newtonian" and "Descartian." Its basic assumption that all disease originates in chemical malfunctions leads to an inclusive analytical deduction of biochemical details. This focus on biochemistry leads to a mountain of details and facts about the body but tends to lose sight of the person as an integrated entity.

The successes are undeniable and impressive—we are not suggesting a return to a simpler era—but the failures and shortcomings are often overlooked, overshadowed by the dazzle of promising new technology and biochemical revelations. Indeed, areas like emergency medicine, surgery, and infectious disease, which lend themselves to biochemical treatment and medical technology have been particularly successful. However, an objective examination of the results of chronic disease treatment reveals few true advances in this area. The incidence of most forms of cancer has risen steadily since the turn of the century when far fewer people died of the disease. In the complex field of cancer treatment, there is much disagreement even within medical professions about the effectiveness of some standard forms of cancer therapy.[16]

Modern medicine has not fared much better in the treatment

of chronic diseases. Diabetes and hypertension can be controlled to some extent by drug therapy, but not cured. Furthermore, the cause of most chronic diseases remains an elusive mystery. If a specific causative factor such as bacteria or virus cannot be implicated, then the cause and cure remain nebulous; the biochemical rationale is routinely applied to all major diseases. Diabetes, arthritis, high blood pressure, cancer, and even emotional/mental disorders are attributed to biochemical disorders.[17] This analytical reduction of all disease processes to chemical imbalance is the great speciality of the biochemical model. It has resulted in brilliant achievements and a very systematic methodology, but is it the total picture, and does it fully account for the spectrum of health and disease? Do these chemicals that constitute our bodies exist in a vacuum where thought, emotions, diet, weather, and social adjustments have little or no influence on health? In the holistic model the causative factor, such as the specific molecule, is not the main objective of diagnosis; rather, the goal is the restoration of equilibrium to the whole organism. This is a very different methodological perspective.

Because of the shortcomings of biochemical medicine, it is the opinion of the authors that the enormous expense of some kinds of medical technology (i.e., organ transplants) would be better served by researching the mystery of degeneration and regeneration. How can we prevent this degeneration in the first place? Even more urgent is the question—what are the factors that lead to immune deficiency? Immune deficiency is possibly responsible for a host of new epidemics: Candida albicans, Epstein-Barr virus, and AIDS. It is suspected that immune deficiency can be caused by abusing recreational drugs and ingesting poor quality food. What role does the abuse of medical drugs play?[18] In the last decades of the twentieth century, the myth that drugs and surgery can eradicate disease is rapidly being undermined.

Where is the biochemical model taking us? Are we truly entering a new age of medicine based on technologies like genetic engineering, or is this direction merely a further elaboration of past models, with the same strengths and limitations? Have we really entered a new age of medical utopia, as some sources would have us believe? This book is not intended to be a criticism of modern medicine, but we would like to question some of its powerful myths. Obviously, great advances have been made in medical science, but there are holes in the facade. Numerous books and articles have described the alarming tendency in modern practice to the intemperate prescription of drugs, polypharmacy (the mixing of many drug therapies in one patient), an excessive use of surgery, and iatrogenic (doctor-caused) disease. Drug- and doctor-dependence are encouraged; self-sufficiency in health is not. Too much medical meddling can create more problems, however, because it overlooks the subtle homeostasis of health and concentrates on the strong-arm tactics of biochemical and surgical intervention. Our present medical science has gained great power over the body. The body's tissues and fluids can be monitored, probed, catheterized, scanned, drugged, anesthethized, radiated, or surgically removed, but is the quality of health really improving? What about the health of a person, his or her well-being and vitality? What about the integrity of the organism? Is *quantity* of life more important than *quality*?

Within the present medical establishment it is presently very difficult to question some of the assumptions of the biochemical model. Because disagreement amounts to heresy and results in professional censure, one rarely finds articles relating, even obliquely, to holistic ideas in standard medical journals. Today, there are many medical doctors interested in bioenergetic medicine, but these are a quiet minority.

The story is told that when Galileo discovered the moons of Jupiter through his newly invented telescope the priests refused to accept his request even to glance through the eyepiece. For them to admit that those moons existed would be tantamount to admitting that their model of the universe was askew. Those Catholic priests were afraid of looking at the evident facts, of having to accept the unknown and being forced to revise their model. The new untoward facts were a threat to their world view, assumptions and dogma. Ironically, we have reached an era in Western civilization when the scientific priests of our technological culture refuse, like the Catholic priests in Galileo's time, to look through the proverbial telescope at the moons of Jupiter.

There is a growing mass of information regarding this life energy, but it has been ignored or derided. The conventional response is that it can't be true, so why examine it? But the true strength of the scientific spirit is first to observe, examine, test, and then to pass judgment. One of the difficulties in examining holistic ideas is that it involves a shift in the way we see. After all, we are all children of Newton and Descartes, and we have been educated to perceive in a certain way: to see parts but not the whole, to specialize, to divide. The science of the future will include the rigorous methodology of science as well as an integrated understanding of the whole.

On the surface the biochemical model is mathematical, neat, and tidy, but the dynamic nature of life and of man tends to undermine this semblance of linear order. Modern science has striven to make medicine into a hard science like chemistry and to avoid the unquantifiable: the emotions, spirit, and subjective sensations. This monumental effort to make medicine into a consistent science solely based on biochemical data tends to disregard the traditional art of healing based on homeostasis and bioenergy. By reducing the human being to an orderly functioning of chemicals, one reduces the unique quality of life, which is greater than he can know with his intellect. Life, after all, consists of mind, body and emotions. Each element contains qualities that cannot easily be quantified. Conversely, there are also limitations in the "Eastern" model which readily sees the larger picture and accepts the bioenergy, but often lacks the inquisitive and analytical drive of its "Western" counterpart.

In conclusion, an acceptance of the holistic perspective involves an understanding of bioenergy, homeostasis, and the integrity of the whole. In this model each person is seen as a unique individual, a complex ecological system of interrelated parts vitalized and regulated by the bioenergy. The three levels of man—body, emotions, and mind—are given careful consideration, but the emotions and mind are recognized as most important in the genesis of disease. Each person is also in vital relationship to the outside environment: climate, family, occupation, society, and cosmic forces. Disease is an expression of imbalance in this complex web of life.

In health the bioenergetic field is balanced and strong. In disease an interference or weakness overcomes the normal vibrational rate of the bioenergy, creating distortions in the field. These distortions or irregularities occur in patterns—a fundamental theme of this book—which are expressed on all levels simultaneously. These patterns are far from nebulous or mystical; they are pragmatic and clinically significant, and the well-trained physician can readily discern them. We call these distortions in the bioenergetic field "patterns of disharmony."[19] The recognition of these patterns of disharmony is the distinguishing characteristic of bioenergetic and holistic medicine.

2

Bioenergetic Research Through History

"Great scientific theories do not usually conquer the world
through being accepted by opponents who, gradually convinced of their truth, have finally adopted them. It is
always rare to find a Saul becoming a Paul. What happens
is that the opponents of the new idea finally die off and
the following generation grows up under its influence."
Max Planck
Nobel Prize Winner in Physics

Introduction

During our studies in Chinese medicine and homeopathy,
we became increasingly amazed at the amount of valid bioenergetical research conducted over the past few centuries. While this
chapter is by no means complete, it is a brief biographical sketch
of the major scientists, physicians, and philosophers throughout
history who have observed and studied this special energy whose
most important and unique feature is the animation of life.

One can't help but ponder why this information is virtually
ignored in the so-called "Age of Reason." On the surface it does
seem puzzling, but an in-depth study reveals the age-old struggle
between vitalism and mechanism. In the last one hundred years,
mechanistic philosophy has for the most part become the law. The
concepts of bioenergy simply do not fit into this present universal
paradigm—the mechanistic, or so-called "Newton-Cartesean,"
model. The stakes are far greater than the average person realizes.
Indeed many a good scientist has had his entire career ruined sim-

ply for researching this taboo subject.

Theories of bioenergy have therefore been discarded or ignored, along with other data that doesn't fit into the mechanistic paradigm. As the pile of discarded data mounts, more and more scientists and philosophers are formulating and expounding new theories in their attempts to explain all of these inconsistencies. It does seem that we are entering a new Renaissance, which Jean Houston, author of *The Possible Human*, lucidly describes as "rhythms of awakening."[1] In view of the information we present in this chapter, we are again reminded of the priest who refused, during the last paradigm shift, to peer through Galileo's telescope at the moons of Jupiter. This time, however, it is the scientists themselves who refuse to look.

3000 B.C.

Huang Ti

The Yellow Emperor, Huang Ti, was the legendary founder of Chinese medicine (circa 3000 B.C.). The first recorded book on Chinese medicine, *The Nei Ching (Inner Classics)*, written in 100 B.C., is a dialogue between Huang Ti and his court physician, Chi Po. The Chinese recognized this concept of bioenergetics thousands of years ago. The simple word *chi* for "life energy" reflects their intrinsic desire for simplicity and harmony.

Prajapati Daksha

Prajapati Daksha is credited as the founder of Ayurvedic medicine, the traditional medicine of India, which is as ancient as Chinese medicine. The Sanskrit word *ayurvedic* means "the science of life."[2] As one might suppose, Ayurvedic practice is similar to its Chinese counterpart in many ways. Its practice includes diet, herbs and medication as well as several types of therapy not used in Chinese medicine, such as gem elixirs. Like Oriental medicine, Ayurvedic medicine is designed to harmonize the pranic energies of the body. For all practical purposes, *chi* and *prana* are identical.

Kahunas

The Kahunas, ancient priests who settled in Hawaii, also developed their own medical system, *Huna* which is based on bioenergetic concepts. The *Huna* term for bioenergy is *mana*.

500 B.C.

Pythagoras of Samos 560–480 B.C.

Little is known of Pythagoras' early life. Born in Greece on the tiny isle of Samos, Pythagoras spent his early years traveling and acquiring knowledge. Although he is better known for his mathematical genius, Pythagoras is also the true father of Hellenic medicine. In fact, Pythagoras was an eclectic, drawing from all areas of knowledge—philosophy, medicine, music, astronomy, mathematics, and esoteric knowledge, to list a few.

Pythagoras considered healing the noblest of all pursuits and spoke often of a healing energy, or *pneuma*. In 529 B.C., the philosopher/physician settled in Crotona, Italy to establish his famous school, the culmination of thirty years of travel and study with the wisest men of Egypt, Chaldea, Persia, Arabia, India, Babylonia and Palestine-Phoenicia. Pythagoras instructed his students in the totality of body, mind and spirit—a holistic dream.

> His students, all carefully chosen, were advised to begin each day with meditation, and there were many exercises for purification of mind and strengthening of will. The curriculum included harmony, music, the dance, gymnastics, proper diet, mathematics, and astronomy. The harmony achieved through music, dance, and numbers, he believed, was imperative to the health of both body and soul.[3]

It is most unfortunate that so much of his information was lost because of the oral teaching traditions of the early Greeks.

Hippocrates of Cos 460–370 B.C.

The father of Western medicine, Hippocrates was a well-known physician of ancient Greece whose wide and varied experiences led him to describe the natural healing force of nature, *vis medicatrix naturae*. He termed this force *physis*.

Although Hippocrates was a vitalist in thought and action, he indirectly set the stage for the mechanistic perception of medicine. His teachings provided the impetus for the separation of science, religion, and philosophy, thus diverging from the holistic approach of his predecessor, Pythagoras, by becoming more specialized.

1500 A.D.

Paracelsus 1493–1541

Born Theophrastus Bombastus von Hohenheim, this Swiss medical genius wrote over fourteen books dealing with alchemy, ethics, philosophy and healing. Paracelsus, an innovative medical pioneer, stands at the pivotal point between modern and ancient medicine. He was an early vitalist who coined the popular term *quintessence* for his concept of bioenergy.

1600

Jan Baptista von Helmont 1579–1644 A.D.

Von Helmont was a Belgian physician who continued the tradition of Paracelsus. He proposed the existence of a pure vital spirit that permeates all of nature, a universal fluid that cannot be weighed or measured. Von Helmont calls this vital spirit *archeus*, a Greek word meaning "idea" or "form." The Chinese have a similar concept, and later Bergson, Driech, and Sheldrake continued with their own modern concepts of idea and form.

Robert Fludd 1574–1637

An English physician who used magnets for healing, Fludd proposed that all life force originates from the sun and is consequently manifested in all living matter. Fludd simply refers to this life force as *the fluid*. Fludd, without any knowledge of the similar Chinese medical philosophy, postulated that this bioenergy enters the body with the breath.

Issac Newton 1642–1727

Isaac Newton's monumental work, *The Principa Mathematica*, is considered the greatest single scientific work in history. In this pivotal book, he presents in great detail the laws of motion and gravity which form the physical basis for what is called "the Newton-Cartesean universal paradigm." Ironically, in the last section of this book Newton freely discusses his personal views concerning a "subtle spirit" found in human bodies. His view of bioenergetics is quite clearly summarized in the concluding paragraph of his immortal book.

> And now we might add something concerning a certain most *subtle spirit*, which pervades and lies hid in all gross bodies; by the force and action of which *Spirit*, the particles of bodies mutually attract one another at near distances, and cohere, if contiguous; and electric bodies operate to greater distances, as well as repelling and attracting the neighboring corpuscles; and light is emitted, reflected, refracted, inflected, and heats bodies; and all sensation is excited, and members of animal bodies move at command of the will, namely, by the vibration of this *Spirit*, mutually propagated along the solid filaments of the nerves, from the outward organs of sense to the brain, and from the brain into the muscles. But these are the things that cannot be explained in few words, nor are we furnished with that sufficiency of experiments which is required to an accurate determination and demonstration of the laws by which this electric and elastic *Spirit* operates.[4]

We should add that René Descartes, the philosophical half of the Newton-Cartesean paradigm, was also a vitalist at heart. On bioenergy, Descartes states:

> Filling the spaces in the nerves is a fine, material substance, the *animal spirit*. These spirits are actually the most quickly moving particles of the blood that have travelled through the arteries in the shortest, straightest path from the heart to the brain. Once conveyed to the brain according to the laws of mechanics and then separated from the coarser parts of the blood, these most agile particles become a wind or very subtle flame.[5]

Descartes' writings on physiology are filled with references to these "winds" and "subtle spirits."

While it is widely known that Newton was a student of the occult, spending much of his later life in the study of astrology, metaphysics, and other spirtual pursuits, few scientific histories mention that Descartes was interested in the Rosicrucian order, a body of esoteric knowledge still active today.[6] Whether he was actually a member is not certain because of his extreme caution (and rightfully so—many of his fellow thinkers, including Galileo, Bruno and Ramus, were imprisoned for heresy).

It is clearly a grave injustice, therefore, to name the mechanistic paradigm after these two free thinkers, either of whom would scoff at the limitations of the mechanistic model. This fact is well documented in literature. To Thomas Huxley's nineteenth-century philosophical defense of mechanistic thought:

> I am prepared to go with the materialists wherever the true pursuit of the path of Descartes may lead them . . . I hold, with the materialist, that the human body, like all living bodies, is a machine, all the operations of which will, sooner or later be explained on physical principles. I believe that we shall, sooner or later, arrive at a mechanical equivalent of consciousness, just as we arrived at a mechanical equivalent of heat.

Twentieth-century Harvard philosophy professor Ralph Eaton replies:

> A mechanical equivalent of consciousness! Descartes would have laughed the phrase aside as meaningless and self-contradictory, as no less absurd than the statement that a straight line could be curved. The soul stands by itself, independent of the world of matter and co-equal with the body it inhabits.[7]

It seems the dream of mechanistic science to disprove the very existence of the soul, or to reduce it to a chemical equation.

1700

George Stahl 1660–1739

Dr. Stahl, a leading German physician and chemist who disdained the use of chemicals for healing, postulated the existence of an intelligent life force which he named *anima*. In his opinion, this anima regulated the body and could be used for healing purposes. His vitalistic teachings were continued throughout the eighteenth and nineteenth centuries at the medical school in Montpellier, France. Interestingly enough, both William Cullen and Samuel Hahnemann were influenced by Stahl.[8] Hahnemann later went on to devise homeopathy, a remarkable bioenergetic medicine.

Samuel Hahnemann 1755–1815

Samuel Hahnemann, the great German physician who discovered the science of homeopathy while translating a medical book by William Cullen, coined one of the most popular terms ever used to describe life energy: *vital force*. Dr. Hahnemann's book, *The Organon of Medicine*, describes his system of bioenergetic medicine in detail and remains essential reading for the aspiring young homeopath of today. In the next chapter on homeopathy we will discuss Hahnemann and his science in greater detail.

Franz Anton Mesmer 1734–1815

Mesmer received his medical doctorate from the University of Vienna. Historically, he is known as the father of hypnosis. Realizing the powerful curative response in Mesmer's forceful bedside manner, his followers, the Société de L'Harmonie Universelle, extended this rapport in the development of the hypnotic phenomenon. Mesmer's real interest, however, was in bioenergetics, which he called *animal magnetism*. Mesmer discovered that this energy could be used for healing and that it could be accumulated and stored in special devices. In his writing, he goes to great length explaining the differences between animal magnetism and ordinary magnetic force.

Luigi Galvani 1737–1798

Dr. Galvani graduated from the University of Bologna, Italy, with degrees in medicine and philosophy. Although anatomy was his true passion, his name is immortalized in the field of electricity for his discovery of electrical current. Many inventions and concepts bear his name: the galvanometer, galvanizing, and galvanic skin resistance, to name a few.

A vitalist at heart, this pioneer in electro-neurophysiology was determined to prove the existence of a bioelectrical energy. Galvani's famous frog-leg experiments, connecting various circuits with several kinds of metals to frog nerves, were the basis for his vitalistic theories. Alessandro Volta, another immortal name of this era, proposed that Galvani's theory of *life force* was in error. He demonstrated that the twitch created in the frog's leg was caused when two dissimilar metals in an electrolytic solution created a current, rather than the hypothesized "animal electricity." Volta later used these concepts to create the storage battery.

It is not so well known that Galvani devised another experiment which excluded all metal from the frog leg, proving the existence of an animal electricity. This work was corroborated by Alexander von Humbolt, but both of these papers were ignored for the same reasons that similar data is ignored today. It is paradoxical to realize that Volta and Galvani were both right. Volta's bi-metallic currents are a fact, but Galvani's theory of a living current has also been proven true—injured flesh produces a measurable "current of injury."[9]

Karl von Reichenbach 1788–1869

The German industrial scientist Karl von Reichenbach obtained his Ph.D. from the University of Tubingen. Early in his career, Reichenbach discovered the organic chemicals paraffin and kreosote, thus assuring his place in history. Later, after starting his own steel foundry, Reichenbach became interested in the study of bioenergetics, which he ornately referred to as *the odic force*. His colleagues were, needless to say, skeptical about his unorthodox research, claiming his theories to be the eccentricity of a great scientist. Mechanistic biographies, resistant to bioenergetic research, attempt to discredit Reichenbach's work by claiming that this meticulous scientist used poor techniques.[10] Nonetheless, he was both ardent and tenacious, sometimes performing a single experiment a hundred times to be absolutely positive his research was valid. Historically, it is interesting to notice how many reputable researchers observed this same phenomenon, independently drawing virtually identical conclusions.

1800

Justus Liebig 1803–1873

Liebig, another German, was a professor of chemisty at the University of Geissen and the University of Munich. A formidable leader in the newly-emerging field of organic chemistry, Liebig is best known for his pioneering work in the field of agricultural chemistry, the study of the chemical processes that regulate plant growth and how chemicals affect that growth. His research led directly to the use of fertilizers for the stimulation of crop growth. Although a major figure in chemistry, he felt that chemicals alone would not explain the phenomena of life.

Chemists could duplicate many organic chemical substances, but because they could not hope to duplicate, for instance, an eye or a leaf, Liebig reasoned that there is "something in life" beyond chemistry that regulates or governs the creation of living forms.

William Gregory 1803–1858

Son of famous Scottish mathematician James Gregory, William Gregory was schooled in medicine and chemistry at the University of Edinburgh, where later he became a well-respected professor. Dr. Gregory, the first researcher to describe the process for refining crude rubber to isoprene, was also involved in the synthesis of morphine and codeine from opium.

Gregory worked with Justus Liebig for four years, translating most of Liebig's work into English. While in Germany, Gregory also became interested in the works of Karl von Reichenbach and translated *The Odic Force* into English. He independently verified Reichenbach's experiments, and, like Reichenbach, Gregory was rejected by his colleagues, who refused to accept this "ridiculous theory." Like many contemporary scientists, Gregory's career was ruined because of his involvement in bioenergetic research.

Hippolyte Baraduc

Dr. Baraduc, a French physician inspired by Reichenbach, once again observed this bioenergy phenomena and linked *la force vitale* to the respiration, corraborating the theories of Robert Fludd as well as those of Chinese medical philosophy. Baraduc also noticed that this force leaves the body at the moment of death, a fact mentioned in his book on his research, *Les Vibrations de la Vitalité Humaine.*

Dr. Luys

Dr. Luys, of the Hospital de la Charité, France, worked in collaboration with psychic researcher Colonel de Rochas. He discovered that the human body is polarized, the right side being positive and the left negative. This observation concurs with the Chinese, who state the right side of the body is *yang* (+) and the left side is *yin* (−).[11]

1900

Walter Kilner 1847–1920

A graduate of Cambridge University, London physician Walter Kilner invented a special screen enabling anyone to view the aura. (It is proposed that this aura is the actual bioenergetic emanation.) This screen consisted of dicyanine, a special dye derived from coal tar, sandwiched between two sheets of plastic. It acted as a filter for this subtle energy by increasing one's ability to see in the ultraviolet range. Kilner calls this aura *the human atmosphere.* His book by the same name is the first English discussion of this phenomenon as if it were fact. Kilner mentions the use of this screen for diagnosing illness, the aura being noticeably weaker around the affected organ(s). Viewing with this screen had the unusual side effect of curing far-sightedness, as reported by Kilner and an associate, Oscar Bagnall.

Rene Prosper Blondot 1849–1930

Prosper Blondot, a reknowned French physics professor from

the University of Nancy, established his reputation in the world of science by validating Maxwell's theories on electromagnetism. An exacting scientist with an uncanny ability to make precise measurements of infinitesimal waveforms, he was the first to measure the emission speeds of x-rays and the speed of an electrical current along a wire.

Dr. Blondot's career plummeted when his continuing research led him into the controversial area of bioenergy. He discovered a new radiation, *n-rays*, named after his home town, Nancy. It was Blondot's claim that these N-rays are emitted from living organisms, as well as certain non-organic sources such as magnets and the sun. At least fourteen of Blondot's associates became involved in this research, publishing various papers and generating much enthusiasm and public attention. The most notable of these colleagues were De Lipinay, reporting N-rays emanating from the soundwaves of tuning forks and sirens; Charpentier, who discovered N-rays to be stronger in well-rested and mentally-active people; and Cleaves, who reasoned that because N-rays were longer than heat waves but shorter than radio waves, they must behave similarly to infrared waves.

It is not fully understood how or why Blondot's work was so completely invalidated. For one, a physics professor at Johns Hopkins University, Robert Wood, published his most unscientific exposé of Blondot in the prestigious science magazine, *Nature*. This exposé attacking Blondot's research is more akin to Wood's hobby, ghost-busting, than to true scientific procedure.[12] The scientific community at that time had a heavily-vested interest in eliminating vitalistic research and were eager to hear Blondot's investigations repudiated. To this day, most people do not appreciate the fact that this subtle bioenergy requires new and radically different investigative procedures. It is a sad note that this brilliant scientist's career was ruined and that his valuable discoveries were allowed to slip by.

Dr. E. Barety

Barety, another French doctor, published his independently-derived research describing *nerve energy*, this "newly-discovered" force. Barety's massive book, *Le Magnetism Animal Etudié sous le Nom de Force Nervique Rayonnante et Circulante*, reiterates much of what has already been detailed by other researchers concerning bioenergetic phenomena.

Albert Abrams 1863–1924

Albert Abrams was one of those rare multi-dimensional geniuses, an expert in many fields. His background is best described by Edward Russell, a Fleet Street editor, in the book, *Report on Radionics:*

> Albert Abrams, A.M., LLD, M.D., was born in San Francisco in 1863 and qualified at an accredited medical college before he was of age or could receive his diploma. He learned German and went to the University of Heidelberg, where he graduated in medicine with the highest possible honors. Still a very young man, he spent a long time doing post-graduate work in Heidelberg, Berlin, Paris, Vienna, and London under such famous teachers as Virchow, Frerichs, Wasserman and Hermann von Helmholtz.
>
> Von Helmholtz, of course, was one of the great scientific figures and teachers of the nineteenth century. He was a physician, a physiologist, a physicist, a mathematician and a philosopher of science. It was first as a pupil and then as a friend of von Helmholtz that Abrams acquired a knowledge of the exciting developments in physics of those days—something unusual in a young doctor.[13]

Abrams proved to be an extraordinary sort of broad-thinking eclectic, synthesizing vast areas of knowledge. He was quite famous and well-respected. Not only did he serve as Dean of Clinical Medicine at Stanford University, but he also managed to write twelve books and numerous papers in many areas of medicine. Like Samuel Hahnemann, Abrams founded a new science, the study of radionics. An attempt to correlate the laws of biology with those of physics, radionics is a science that studies the subtle emanations from life forms and how they apply to the diagnosis and treatment of disease. Abrams claimed that there is not just one, but rather three distinct types of emanations. In one of his more esoteric books, *New Concepts in Diagnosis and Treatment,* Abrams describes these emanations as *physical energy, psychical energy,* and *auric energy.*

1900

Emile Boirac

Rector of the Academy at Dijon, France, Boirac was a leading philosopher and psychologist who presided several times over the International Congress of Experimental Psychology. Boirac became interested in bioenergy, which he refers to by the name *nerve radioactivity.* In his book *Our Hidden Forces,* Boirac emphatically states:

> In my frank opinion, magnetic radio-action or nerve radioactivity exist as palpably as the radioactivity of light and heat; and I am firmly convinced that, whosoever will experiment in observing the condition which I did, if he be possessed with sufficient patience, will reach the same conclusion.[14]

Boirac also discusses the ability of one organism to affect another over a distance through this radioactivity.

These experiments by Boirac were stimulated by the early works of Ambroise Liebault, a French physician, whose experiments with children indicated that one organism could affect another over a distance. The results of both were later confirmed by S. Alrutz, a Swedish researcher. Alrutz states, "One nervous system can exert a direct influence upon another through a distance."[15]

Henri Bergson 1859–1941

Henri Bergson was the French philosopher who posits his famous vitalistic hypothesis of *élan vital* in such popular works as *Time and Free Will, Matter and Memory,* and *Creative Evolution.* Bergson's philosophy gave rise to a resurgent interest in vitalism, but due to a lack of sophisticated tools for measurement of this energy, it appeared that vitalism had once and for all been laid to rest.

Hans Driesch 1867-1941

Prominent German embryologist Hans Driesch, who received his doctorate at the University of Jena, was a confirmed vitalist. Strongly opposed to the mechanistic view dominating embryology during his lifetime, Driesch thought that physio-chemical processes could not entirely account for the vast complexities of organic regulation, regeneration and reproduction; machines simply don't reproduce. This, he felt, was the blindspot in the mechanistic view. Driesch proposes his concept, *entelechy*, a non-energetic field influencing form. Entelechy, not precisely identical to *chi*, is more closely related to *li*, another Chinese concept discussed in detail with regard to Rupert Sheldrake's hypothesis of morphogenetic fields (mentioned in the first chapter and later in this chapter).

Driesch, believing that the action of enzymes was somehow instrumental in this process of entelechy, strongly emphasized the importance of enzymes as regulating agents for biological development. Later, Russian scientist Alexander Gurvich added even more weight to this hypothesis.

W.E. Boyd

W.E. Boyd, M.A., M.D., continued the work of Albert Abrams in this new science of radionics. Boyd, another innovative thinker, invented his own radionic device, calling his machine the Emanometer (after human emanations).

In an unprecedented trial, the Royal Society of Medicine attempted once and for all to end the outlandish claims for these little black radionic boxes. Lord Horder, head of the Society, singled out for demonstration Dr. Boyd's Emanometer, but much to his chagrin, the Emanometer passed twenty-five separate tests with 100% accuracy. For this to happen by chance would be astronomical: 1 to 33,554,432. The Horder report was published in the *British Medical Journal* and the *Lancet*, January 25, 1925, but was all too quickly forgotten. No one really wanted to accept its extraordinary implications.

Paul Kammerer 1880–1926

An Austrian biologist, Paul Kammerer was opposed to Gregor Mendel's genetic theory. Mendel's theory claims that genetic change occurs only through natural selection and random mutation of genes on a purely chemical physiological basis. Kammerer was a proponent of the opposing camp, the Lamarckian genetic theory which postulates that environmental influences could be inherited. Supporting vitalistic views, Kammerer spoke often of an organic-based life force which he called *formative energy*. In the scientific climate of his day, his research and ideas made no impact, and up to this day, Darwin and Mendel's mechanistic view of evolution has remained unchanged.

1930

Korshet and Ziegler

Korshet and Ziegler were two German research scientists who discovered that certain metals, such as copper, emit vitalizing radiations, while others, such as lead, emit devitalizing radiations. This discovery is the inspiration for the works of physicist Oscar Brunler (whose biography appears later in this chapter).

Fritz Grunewald

A German electrical engineer, Fritz Grunewald, demonstrated that man's body is comprised of a complicated magnetic field with many magnetic centers. The Ayurvedic physicians of India have taught this for centuries, calling the larger magnetic centers *chakras*, and the smaller ones *nadis*. These centers appear to form lines or pathways through the body similar to acupuncture points and meridians.

Erich Muller

A Swiss geophysicist and engineer from Zurich, Erich Muller discovered a subtle emanation coming from the living body. He not only photographed these emanations but determined that they can be conducted along nonconductors such as silk, paper, wood and glass. Paralleling the Chinese concepts of *chi*, Muller's research showed that these emanations are affected by activity, drugs, respiration, and radiate most intensely at the fingertips.

W. Guyon Richards

Richards, a distinguished London surgeon and administrator, used radionic equipment to detect ring-like concentric life forces around human beings. Richards named these rings *biomorphs*. Later, Dr. Harold Burr of Yale University provided further evidence of these life fields using more standard scientific equipment.

Harold Burr

Burr, a prominent professor of anatomy and neuroanatomy for forty-three years at Yale University School of Medicine, was considered one of the top neuroanatomists and embryologists in the world. Burr's book *Blueprint for Immortality* was the culmination of his years as a top researcher in the field of bioenergetic phenomena. Burr states, "The result of these many years of experimentation leave no reasonable doubt that the field characteristics of a living system is a basic property of life."[16] During this work Burr and his close associates, colleagues and friends (such as F.S.C. Northrup, philosopher; Dr. Henry Margenau, physicist; Dr. Eugene Higgins, Professor of Physics and Natural Philosophy at Yale; and Dr. Leonard Ravitz, M.D.) repeatedly renamed this field: from "electro-magnetic" to "electro-dynamic," to "electro-static," to "quasi electro-static," and finally "life fields" or, more simply *L-fields*. Burr clarifies:

> It does not make any difference whether you call it an electrostatic field, an electro-magnetic field, or an electro-dynamic field. The name is always a consequence of the methods which were applied to its study. In other words, there is one unifying characteristic of the Universe which we have ignored, and that is its field properties.[17]

Burr went on to postulate that these L-fields act as blueprints for the development of living organisms, and that through these fields we are interconnected with the entire universe. It is most unfortunate that this extremely valuable work was considered by his mechanistic colleagues to be but foggy vitalism.

Leonard Ravitz

Dr. Ravitz, a scientist and physchiatrist from Yale University, discovered that human emotion produces a measurable effect in the electro-dynamic field of the body. These effects can be measured in the millivolt range. Ravitz's work was held in high esteem by Dr. Harold Burr.

Alexander Gurvich 1874–1954

A Russian scientist, Alexander Gurvich, discovered that all living cells produce an invisible radiation, which he called *mitogenic radiation*. Gurvich determined that muscle tissue, cornea, blood and nerves are all transmitters of this special energy. Gurvich observed the release of this energy during enzymatic reactions, reinforcing Hans Driesch's theory that enzymes were somehow instrumental to this process.

Dr. and Madame Margrou

A husband-and-wife team at the Pasteur Institute in Paris, Dr. and Madame Margrou discovered that radiation from living tissue can be used to affect the growth of plant rootlets and bacteria.[18]

Otto Rahn

Professor of Bacteriology at Cornell University, Rahn claimed that the invisible radiations of living organisms are of considerable physiological significance. Not only do they play a distinct part in cell division and growth; most likely, they also govern the healing process.[19]

Wilhelm Reich 1887–1957

Reich received his medical degree from the University of Vienna. Afterwards, he became a student of Sigmund Freud. Eventually these two great men parted ways over a difference in opinion on clinical application. In his desire to prove that love and life are but electrical flows, Reich once again discovered the phenomenon of bioenergy. Reich called this energy *orgone*. He theorized that emotional trauma, especially of a sexual nature, creates muscle tension which he termed "armoring." This armoring prevents the free flow of orgone through the body. By freeing this body of armor, Reich felt that the emotional nature of the patient would improve.[20]

Further research in this field of bioenergy led Reich to discover methods of accumulating and utilizing this energy. Reich began using orgone accumulators for the successful treatment of various disorders, including cancer. The FDA refused to allow the sale of these accumulators and eventually incarcerated him for the illegal sales. Quite possibly, these attacks on Reich were generated by the prevailing McCarthy-era atmosphere and by the bias against bioenergetic research. After his incarceration, all of Reich's works were burned in a public incinerator. Shortly thereafter, he died from a heart attack, probably the result of seeing his life's work destroyed. However, Reich's tremendous intellect and spirit did not disappear without leaving a distinct ripple in the world of psychology and healing, and his influence is once again strong in America.

Silvester Prat and Jan Schlemmer

Two Czechoslovakian researchers, Prat and Schlemmer, captured on film an unusual radiation originating from living tissue. They observed that this radiation could penetrate xylonite, a material which is impermeable to infrared, ultraviolet and visible radiation. Their research, a precursor to the development of the more popular Kirlian photographs, indicated that this radiation was a new form of energy.

1940

Aubrey Westlake 1893–

Dr. Westlake was originally introduced to radionics after the successful treatment of a problem unresolved by orthodox methods. A prominent London physician turned radionics practitioner, he collaborated with E. Eeman to determine that bioenergy flows along definite pathways, a study that supports Chinese meridian theory. Dr. Westlake retired in 1984 at the age of ninety-one.

I.I. Rabi

With his associates at Columbia University, P. Kurch and S. Millman, Rabi demonstrated that each living cell behaves like a tiny radio transmitter (and receiver) emitting a continuous broadcast over the entire range of the electro-magnetic spectrum.

George de la Warr

George de la Warr was an English engineer whose resumé includes: chief engineer assistant for an oil refinery, chief constructional engineer for Firestone Rubber, and development engineer for Firestone Rubber. De la Warr lifted the science of radionics to new heights, devising some of the finest pieces of radionics equipment ever produced. All his life de la Warr was fascinated by fine instruments; consequently, he was exacting of the tools he purchased or constructed.

With his wife, de la Warr produced volumes of works on radionics. They showed how the principles of radionics could be used in both veterinarian and agricultural applications—in short, on all living forms. Radionics was used in 1949 by Curtis Upton for the successful treatment of vegetable crops in Pennsylvania against insects. These experiments were observed by B.A. Rockwell, director of research for the Pennsylvania Farm Bureau Co-Operative. His conclusion that "radionic treatments are more effective than chemicals" was hushed by the upper echelon of the U.S. Agriculture Department.[21] Rumor has it that this action was stimulated by the lobbying efforts of certain chemical companies.

The de la Warrs, now deceased, organized the Radionic Association of Great Britain. It is still active and thriving in England today.

1950

Oscar Brunler

Dr. Brunler, a California physician and physicist, was inspired by the research of Korschivelt and Ziegler. Brunler discovered *dielectric biocosmic energy*, which he felt is the clue to explaining the auric phenomena. Brunler's book, *Rays and Radiation*, extensively discusses his views concerning bioenergetics.

H.H. Kritzinger

Kritzinger, a German doctor from Dusseldorf, once again confirmed the existence of human emanations. He emphasized that this radiation is strongly dependent on weather conditions and changes in the condition of the air. Not only do his experiments verify the ancient Chinese concepts of environmentally-caused disease, but provide us with a much more reliable source than the recent English experiment using artificially-stimulated weather conditions. This experiment erroneously concluded that weather has no effect on acute diseases. Weather is, in fact, more than a mechanically produced phenomena; it is the range of electromagnetic (and undiscovered) energies that accompany and catalyze it, making it virtually impossible to reproduce under laboratory conditions.

Hans Selye 1907–

Among the greatest modern-day researchers, Selye received his medical degree from Prague University in Germany. Selye holds doctorates in medicine, philosophy and science, as well as nineteen honorary degrees from universities around the world. Dr. Selye has served as professor and Director of Experimental Medicine and Surgery at the University of Montreal since 1945. In addition, he has written over thirty-two books as well as more than 1500 technical articles.

Hans Selye, through his extensive research, has come to recognize a quality of life which he cautiously terms *adaptive energy*.

This energy, he feels, is a basic feature of life itself. Selye, who never actively aligned himself with vitalism, hints that adaptive energy can be experimentally verified. Adaptive energy, however, remains a hypothesis which he suggests will have a great impact on health and medicine.

1960

Hiroshi Motoyama

Hiroshi Motoyama, who received his doctorate in philosophy and psychology at Tokyo University, has additionally studied and practiced acupunture for twenty years, serving as an advisor for the Japanese Acupuncture Association. Motoyama, also an inventor, developed many pieces of electronic equipment for the detection and measurement of the energy fields in man, and over the years he has amassed an incredible wealth of information in all areas of life energy research. He calls this force *ki* (pronounced "key") in the Japanese tradition. Motoyama has written numerous technical books, for example: *How to Measure and Diagnose the Functions of the Meridians and the Corresponding Internal Organs;* and *The Ejection of Energy from the Chakra's of Yogi and the Meridian Points of Acupuncture.*

Robert Miller

A top industrial research scientist with a doctorate in chemical engineering, Miller has written many articles on topics such as metallurgy, high polymers and fluid flow. Miller, inspired by quantum physics, used an atomic cloud chamber to measure human emanations which he eloquently termed *paraelectricity.* Dr. Miller has actually derived a specific formula for determining an individual's bioenergy. This energy is measured in units of "Worralls," named after Ambrose Worrall, the aircraft engineer and psychic healer. Worrall, who died in 1972, assisted Miller until his death. Dr. Miller suggests that this paraelectricity is synonymous with *chi, prana, odic force, orgone,* and the *life fields* of Burr.

Semyon Kirlian

Kirlian and his wife Valentina are the famous Russian research team who developed the interesting but controversial technique for photographing the aura of living organisms known as Kirlian photography. The technique, while producing interesting visual phenomena, has not yet convinced the majority of scientists of its validity.

Y. Inyushin (et al)

A group of Soviet scientists working with Kirlian photography announced their 'new' discovery: all living matter—plants, animals, and humans—not only have a physical body comprised of atoms and molecules, but also a counterpart body comprised of energy, *the biological plasma body.*

1970

Dolores Krieger 1921–

Krieger, Ph.D., R.N., and Professor of Nursing at New York University, is the author of the well-known book on the phenomena of healing entitled *The Therapeutic Touch.* A course by this same name is now taught to nurses and lay people interested in healing. Dr. Krieger, noted for her research demonstrating the validity of the bioenergetic healing phenomena, observed under strict laboratory conditions how therapeutic touch raises hemoglobin levels in test subjects.

John Pierrakos and Alexander Lowen

Pierrakos is a highly esteemed psychiatrist who studied with Wilhelm Reich. Pierrakos and his associate Alexander Lowen, M.D., have developed their own system of therapy based on Reichian thought—known as "bioenergetics"—which is propagated through their Institute of Bioenergetic Analysis.

Pierrakos, freely testifying to his ability to read auras, supports Abrams' claim that not one but three fields of energy surrounds man. In numerous articles, Pierrakos has thoroughly described these fields as he sees and understands them. Dr. Pierrakos is well respected for his uncanny accuracy in diagnostics.

Marcel Vogel

Marcel Vogel retired in 1984 after twenty-seven years as a Senior Research Scientist for IBM. Vogel's San Jose home is filled with awards for his many diverse discoveries in fields such as optics, magnetics and liquid crystals. Best known for developing the magnetic coating used on computer discs, he later became interested in plant research. Vogel hypothesizes a life force which surrounds all living matter. He feels that certain sensitive people can attune themselves to this energy field and, through this field, elicit responses in plants as well as create a climate for healing in animals. Vogel's series of experiments demonstrating that mind energies could be focused and received by a philodendron leaf and registered as a charge in millivolts on a chart recorder literally changed the direction of his life. He has gone on to discover that quartz crystal can be used to amplify healing energies in much the same manner that the crystal in a laser can be used to organize light into a cohesive wave front. Quartz crystal can also directly interact with this healing energy. For several years, Vogel has been spending his retirement teaching medical doctors and other healthcare professionals (including the authors) the use of crystals for accelerating healing.

Vogel is currently researching the role of water structure in healing. He believes that it is possible to identify homeopathic remedies and potencies accurately with existing high-tech instrumentation.

Thelma Moss

Dr. Thelma Moss, a researcher who formerly worked at UCLA, has independently investigated the works of Inyushin and Kirlian. She has developed her own techniques for making these photographs, including a method for producing them in color. Moss speculates that this phenomenon is the same invisible energy system described in ancient Chinese and Indian texts as *chi* and *prana.*

William Tiller

Born in Canada, Dr. Tiller is Chairman of Materials Engineering at Stanford University and the author of over 100 scientific papers. Tiller's studies of Kirlian, Inyushin and other areas of bioenergetic research (which he calls *psycho-energetics*) has led him to the conclusion that the present universal paradigm is in need of expansion. According to Tiller, Einstein did not invalidate Newton, but rather expanded upon Newton's knowledge, just as others will expand upon Einstein's knowledge. Science is a living, growing field.

Tiller refers to five basic areas of data which are not presently covered by the mechanistic paradigm, yet are in need of explanation:[22]

1. Energy fields that are completely different from those known to conventional science.

2. Phenomena which follow a different path than the usual space-time framework.

3. Phenomena that violate the second law of thermodynamics (entropy).

4. Radiation patterns or holograms of energy that act as force envelopes for the organization of substance on a physical level.

5. Evidence that at some level all substance in the universe is interconnected.

There are unexplained data accumulated in all five of these categories. As this Dr. Tiller states:

> We may liken conventional scientific understanding of the universe to the visible tip of an iceberg. We have come to know that exposed tip fairly well. However, most of nature is still hidden from us and we know it not. History contains references and speculation to many aspects of the hidden iceberg and very recent research . . . suggest[s] some fascinating characteristics.[23]

1980

Rupert Sheldrake

After obtaining a Ph.D. in biology from Cambridge, Sheldrake's career led him to the International Research Institute in India where he served as their Consultant Plant Physiologist. In his book, *A New Science of Life,* Sheldrake has formulated an exciting new hypothesis, which he calls "formative causation." This hypothesis proposes that living organisms and all non-living substances form, develop and behave according to what he terms *morphogenetic fields.* Sheldrake, obviously inspired by Paul Weiss (who coined the term "morphogenetic"), is also influenced by vitalists such as Driesch, Bergson, and others. He insists, however, that the important difference in his theory is its total separation from previous vitalistic concepts such as *entelechy, vital force, chi, bioenergy* and the rest. Formative causation addresses the phenomenon of formation without attempting to explain how it works. Sheldrake neither adheres to nor denies vitalistic concepts; rather, he introduces the evidence for his theory, purposely avoiding the bioenergetic controversy. As can be seen from the diverse reactions to his book in the scientific community, this step in itself was tantamount to mutiny. Sheldrake indicates that when formative causation is proven, scientists can begin unravelling its mysteries.

In their explanation of *chi,* the Chinese speak of a similar concept to morphogenetic fields—*li,* which translates "to govern." Chu Hsi, a famous Taoist philosopher of the Twelfth Century, states: "In the Universe there are *li* and *chi.* The *li* is 'what is above shapes' and is the source from which all things are produced. The *chi* is 'what is within shapes' and is the means by which all things are produced."[24]

Sheldrake's concept of morphogenetic fields also contains overtones of Carl Jung's "collective unconscious." Sheldrake presents several new versions of these familiar themes; for instance, he demonstrates that non-living substances such as crystal formations follow a previously unnoticed (or ignored) natural law. Recently, with the proliferation of new chemicals being discovered every year, scientists have noticed a curious fact: The first attempts to crystallize a new chemical from solution is extremely difficult— as if it were trying to decide what form to take—but once the form is chosen, this crystallization process happens with greater ease, even in laboratories thousands of miles away.

Robert Becker

Dr. Becker, an orthopedic surgeon who began his illustrious career at the VA hospital in Syracuse, New York, is a pioneer in the field of tissue regeneration. It would be impossible to list all of Becker's achievements here, but we will mention a few. First of all, he is well known for the use of electricity to heal non-unions in bone fractures. This technique is rapidly gaining popularity in hospitals. He has also discovered a method for using free silver ions as a topical bactericide.

Other discoveries include: the induction of anesthesia using powerful magnetic fields, considerable new information of value in the treatment of cancer, and current investigations into the vitally important new field of electromagnetic pollution (the effect of radio, radar, and microwaves, on the human body).

Of particular interest to the authors is Becker's work with acupuncture. He theorizes that acupuncture meridians are electrical conductors, and the acupuncture points, amplifiers. With the help of a talented biophysicist, he was able to prove a great deal of this theory before their grant was mysteriously cancelled.

Nonetheless, all of the above research stems from his true passion, his primary research—tissue regeneration. Becker has demonstrated the regeneration of a rat's limb from just below its shoulder to its wrist. If Becker had managed this significant feat with biochemical drugs, his name would be a household word. While struggling to understand the unusual results of his experimentation, he has uncovered some startling phenomena. Mammals (rats) have the ability to reconnect and heal severed segments of intestines laid loosely in the abdominal cavity and closed. Strangely enough, these intestines heal even better than controls which were stitched together.

Even more incredible, a salamander with half of his heart gone will completely regenerate a new heart in six hours. Becker feels that this and other regeneration phenomena are controlled and regulated by bioelectrical currents. He has laboratory evidence to support this argument, yet these easily proven facts are ignored and their clinical implications remain unfulfilled.

Becker's determination to uncover the secrets of tissue regeneration with the intention of applying them to medicine has led him into a sensitive fringe area: the study of bioenergy. This research was not calculated to antagonize his fellow scientists, but by their reaction, you would almost think so. In a private communication Becker states, ". . . my main interest over the years has been to evaluate the possible relationships between electromagnetic energy and living things. In no way was I searching for 'the secret of life'; I just believed that the biochemical and reductionist concepts were incomplete and I believe that I have produced some evidence for this idea."

The inescapable direction of his work was simply the necessary result of unbiased exploration into reality. What he has seen in the laboratory cannot be explained entirely by biochemistry (as was suspected all along by great minds such as Liebig and Driesch).

Although a whole new world has been opened for Becker, the reaction from his colleagues has been appalling. Rather than approaching his work with open minds, they choose to react with hostility, derision, namecalling, and worse. What a shock this has been to Becker, naive of the bioenergy prejudice. Becker himself has expressed the indignation he felt when his first innocuous research proposal was met with such acute resistance:

> I had the momentary thrill of imagining myself as Galileo
> or Giordano Bruno; I thought of walking to the window to see
> if the stake and fagots were set up on the lawn. Instead, I de-
> livered a terse speech to the effect that I still thought my hypothe-
> sis was stoutly supported by some very good research, and that
> I was sorry if it flew in the face of dogma. I ended by saying
> that I didn't intend to withdraw the proposal, so they would have
> to act upon it.[25]

Reluctantly, Becker was allowed to begin this initial project which would ultimately draw him to conclude there was more to medicine than biochemistry.

It is unfortunate that his brilliant line of research has been stopped. One has to question the motivation of our scientific establishment when pioneers like Becker are stifled. This strange turn of events, the latest casualty of bioenergetic research, is lucidly explained in his highly recommended book, *The Body Electric.*

Bjorn Nordenstrom 1920–

Dr. Nordenstrom, born in Ragunda, Sweden, and educated at the University of Uppsala, has all the potential for becoming a major name in modern medicine. It is highly likely that Nordenstrom will be credited in Western history with the discovery of the energy circulation system just as Harvey (another vitalist) is credited with that of the blood circulation system. However, the Chinese were aware of both of these facts, and applying them centuries before the West.

Even before this discovery, Nordenstrom had already established an excellent reputation for himself in the field of radiology. He was the pineer of percutaneous needle biopsy, used in every major hospital in the world; radio-opaque chemical dyes; and balloon catheterization for x-raying the heart, blood vessels, and lungs. Not satisfied with these achievements, Nordenstrom was motivated by his deep thirst for understanding the basis of healing and life to undertake an unusual path of research. As early as 1950, Nordenstrom became aware of electrical currents originating in the body and intuitively understood their importance in regulating all types of poorly-understood bodily activities including healing. In 1979, after 30 years of study and research, he felt that at last he truly understood these tiny currents and began the tedious task of compiling this data into his revolutionary book, *Biologically Closed Electrical Circuits: Clinical, Experimental, and Theoretical Evidence for an Additional Circulatory System.* Nordenstrom claims that he has proven the reality of bioelectrical circuits in the body, emphatically stating:

> When you have found all the elements that correspond to
> an ordinary electric circuit, and each element performs its de-
> fined function, it must work.[26]

Nordenstrom goes on to describe how these circuits are switched
on by injury, infection, or tumor. These voltages, it seems, build
and fluctuate in intimate association with the blood vessels, providing the guiding framework for metabolic processes throughout
the body.

> This electrical system, says Nordenstrom, works to balance
> the activity of internal organs and, in the case of injuries, repre-
> sents the very foundation of the healing process. In his view, it's
> as critical to the well-being of the human body as the flow of
> blood. Disturbances in this electrical network, he suggests, may
> be involved in the development of cancer and other diseases.[27]

Rather than just theoretical, Nordenstrom's research has been applied to healing lung cancer victims. In fact, Nordenstrom is developing a reputation for treating otherwise incurable tumors.

Dr. Nordenstrom, like many others in the emerging field of
bioenergy, speculates that his research accounts for acupuncture and
other unexplainable phenomena. Following this train of thought,
a science writer comments:

> Nordenstrom doesn't spare his medical colleagues from the
> jab of his needles. To him, their attitude toward electricity in
> the human body is almost medieval. Knowing of the enormous
> importance of closed electrical circuits in modern electronic
> technology, asks Nordenstrom in the conclusion of the book, is
> it seriously plausible that biology can "afford to ignore" the ex-
> ceedingly efficient principle of transporting electric energy over
> closed circuits?[28]

In closing this section, we should again mention the two apparent directions of bioenergy research: those who examine it as
a type of electro-magnetic phenomena, and those who examine
it as a distinct phenomenon. It is our belief that while aspects of
this energy can be explained in mechanistic electrical terms, when
viewed in its totality, bioenergy must be recognized as different

from ordinary electricity. Bioenergy has a life of its own—a consciousness—apart from electricity.

Conclusion

> "We may ask: If living organisms are composed of molecules that are intrinsically inanimate, why is it that living matter differs so radically from nonliving matter, which also consists of intrinsically inanimate molecules? Why does the living organism appear to be more than the sum of its inanimate parts? The medieval philosopher would have answered that living organisms are endowed with a myterious and divine life-force. But this doctrine, called vitalism, is nothing more than superstition and it has been rejected by modern science. Today it is the basic goal of biochemistry to determine how the collections of inanimate molecules that constitute living organisms interact with each other to maintain and perpetuate the living state."[29]
>
> *Biochemistry*
> Albert Lehninger
> (Johns Hopkins University
> School of Medicine)

This statement on the second page of a popular college biochemistry text succinctly expresses the typical attitude opposing bioenergetic research. What is the reason for this attitude? To answer this complex question requires the utmost objectivity. It is most difficult to refrain from polarizing on a particular side of this timeless question: Is there a living force that animates the body? This controversial theme, recurrent throughout medical history, is presently rejected by the scientific community at large.

Let us examine this issue. On one hand, we have what is called the "establishment." This establishment always champions the currently-accepted knowledge and historically, has always been resistant to new ideas, especially when they directly contradict their favored theories. Historian Daniel Boorstin's description of this resistance seems every bit as accurate today:

At the end of the fifteenth century, any physician who had labored to learn the academic languages and had become the disciple of some professor of medicine had a heavily vested interest in the traditional lore and the accepted dogmas . . . To attack this citadel demanded a willingness to defy the canons of respectability, to uproot oneself from the university community and the guild.[30]

Like all new ideas throughout history, the theory of bioenergy has been met with strong opposition. As Bjorn Nordenstrom has grown to realize: "People who have learned something as truth don't particularly like to hear that they've based a large part of their career on things that were either incomplete or not completely correct."[31] Or as Robert Becker, who has suffered a great deal more injustice, divulges:

I've taken the trouble to recount my experience in detail for two reasons. Obviously, I want to tell people about it because it makes me furious. More important, I want the general public to know that science isn't run the way they read about in the newspapers and magazines.

. . . The present system is in effect a dogmatic religion with a self-perpetuating priesthood dedicated to preserving the current orthodoxies. The system rewards the sycophant and punishes the visionary to a degree unparalleled in the four hundred year history of modern science.[32]

It would seem to the idealist that scientists and medical men would be the most openminded of people, always ready to look at new ideas and to explore. But certainly, it is easy to look at the obvious failings of Western science and criticize. However, we ask, are bioenergetic theories the dogma of tomorrow? What are we doing today to protect the visionary of the future?

Look at the tragic wake bioenergetic research left behind. Galvani died penniless and brokenhearted, while Volta grew rich and famous. Blondot was disgraced and discredited before his fellow scientists and countrymen; this blow to their national scientific credibility took years for the French to recover. Reichenbach, though financially secure, was referred to as an eccentric, while his corraborator and translator, William Gregory (famous in his own right) was ruined by his involvement with bioenergy. Reich died in prison, his life's work burned; and, around the same time, Harold Burr was dismissed as a foggy vitalist. Rupert Sheldrake's book, *A New Science of Life*, was reviewed by *Nature* as "the best candidate for burning there has been for many years." It is ironic that this same magazine, a bastion of modern science, was the very one which, a century earlier, published Robert Wood's unscrupulous exposé of Blondot. In recent times, bioenergetic researchers such as Nordenstrom are routinely ignored unless, like Robert Becker, they make waves so large that the Department of Defense must shut them down. Remarkable men such as these almost never received the recognition they deserve, but, to the contrary: derision, ridicule, and scorn for their efforts; and, unless we can devise a truly equitable system, this is the *status quo*. We support Robert Becker in his statement, "I want our citizens, nonscientists as well as investigators, to work to change the way research is administered. The way it is currently funded and evaluated, we are learning more and more about less and less . . ."[33]

For the last three hundred years, mechanization has reigned supreme, growing into a massive accumulation of technology and knowledge, the like of which early man could not possibly dream. Mechanization, we must realize, has been a necessary path towards true understanding of our universe. Now, as the tide turns, we enter what appears to be a new cycle of history. But, looking back a moment, Pythagoras and others prior to the Renaissance taught that science, religion and philosophy were one. As these teachings evolved, others such as Hippocrates realized the need to divide them in order to gain better insight. It was this thrust that led us into our present age when science, religion and philosophy are separated. That this separation was necessary is unquestionable. For civilization to have developed, this division appears to be an inevitable step.

Coming full circle with the rhythms of civilization, brings to mind the words of Rene Descartes, "Sometimes it is necessary to separate to study but one must ultimately always return to the whole for true understanding." This is the new trend in science.

Bartalanffy's *General System Theory* expresses a need for less specialization and more unity between all sciences. Cybernetics, a computer concept for linking vast areas of information, exemplifies this idea of unity. And now, after a three hundred year cycle of separation, we are witnessing this grand reunion. A similar sentiment is expressed in the book *The Ultimate Frontier:*

> The Western world, and particularly the United States, is entering a second renaissance. The first (during the 15th through 17th centuries) gave rise to scientific methods and led to freedom from religious despotism. This new renaissance is *combining* science and religion as a result of the discoveries of physicists, archeologists, and anthropologists who have found that the knowledge of ancient peoples and many religious traditions contain *facts* of history and the nature of existence. This synthesis is now resulting in people turning from blind religious faith (or no faith) to reasoned belief.[34]

It appears that the general theme of this new renaissance is one of merging: the general system theory merging the sciences; sciences merging with religion and philosophy; left brain merging with right brain; and on a global scale, the East merging with the West.

The purpose of this book is thus threefold. The original intention was to reveal our theories concerning Chinese medicine and homeopathy. Are there natural laws linking them? Do these laws have clinical or philosophical applications? From these questions arose a need to establish the validity and common ground of bioenergy. And then, much more slowly came the realization that we were not opposed to Western medicine (or mechanistic thought) but instead compelled, as we explain in the first chapter, to urge the merging of bioenergetic medicines with the biochemical. Although at times it may seem we are critical of Western medicine, our issues are only with its weak points. It is time for Western medicine to move forward, expanding the biochemical to include the bioenergetic.

This mysterious phenomenon, bioenergy, is profoundly disconcerting to the pragmatic Western mind. For one, not all observers seem equally capable of studying it. Does this mean it does not exist? In *Our Hidden Forces*, Emile Boirac discusses his concept of "cryptodial phenomena," phenomena not yet explainable through the known laws of nature. Boirac reminds us that x-rays did not suddenly begin their existence with the development of tools sensitive enough for their measure; they were always there. Fifty years later, George de la Warr observes:

> For some time it was thought unlikely that any radiation could exist with a higher energy than gamma-rays [gamma rays are higher than x-rays], but at length physicists began to notice something unaccountable was happening to their electroscopes.[35]

This phenomenon was determined by Professor Millikan to be cosmic rays. Cosmic rays are *now* considered by scientists to be the highest energy "possible." But, on the forefront of science is speculation over the existence of the "tachyon," a particle which moves faster than the speed of light.

Understanding the necessity for using sensitive equipment to study bioenergy, Robert Miller opted for an atomic cloud chamber, probably the most sensitive physical tool to date. Others, such as Shafica Karagrulla, a well-known psychiatrist, claim that we are evolving a new sense, enabling the visual perception of bioenergy. Is there radiation beyond cosmic rays? Are there spectrums beyond the electromagnetic? These questions we cannot yet answer. However, there is a real phenomenon, yet unclassified, that science must recognize and begin to study—bioenergy.

Because bioenergetic research deals with such uniquely sensitive energies, its investigations must be innovative and sympathetic to the inherent problems of this study. It is highly likely that thoughts themselves can influence test results, both negatively and positively. Similarly, testing of bioenergetic medicines must observe basic experimental principles and laws or the tests cannot be assumed fair. These medicines, because they deal with totalities and patterns, are highly individualized and do not readily lend themselves to the routine testing techniques of biochemical medicine. A great deal of thought and understanding must go into the proper testing of this energy and its medicines, but these tests are essential if they are ever to become part of the mainstream. (With these thoughts in mind, we have presented in this chapter only researchers with impeccable credentials to substantiate bio-energy. Many researchers who did excellent work were left out for this academic reason.)

While compiling these biographies, it became clear to us how similar these studies were, in spite of the fact that the researchers were sometimes separated by continents and centuries, and often, because of obscurity, unaware of other efforts in the field. This is true even today. In Tables 1 and 2 we summarize the basic properties of bioenergy and list the various synonyms used for this force.

Even into the twentieth century, few, if any, Western investigators were aware of the Chinese or Ayurvedic systems which had developed bioenergy to a sophisticated science long before the onset of Western technological science. Today, we routinely hear doctors such as Nordenstrom and Becker using their discoveries to validate acupuncture. But who is actually validating whom? Physicist Fritjof Capra states that the ancient Chinese masters had special insight into the true nature of the universe that we, in the West, are just now beginning to comprehend. The Oriental knowledge of *chi* far exceeds our limited and superficial understanding of this life energy. By way of analogy, it is like comparing the knowledge of an electrical engineer to that of an electrician.

Meanwhile, evidence of bioenergy continues to mount, and it is clear that the new trend in medicine is toward bioenergetics. Those who fail to see this are reminded that there are still people who believe, in spite of the evidence, that the world is flat. In response to the compelling current of the ensuing new era, physicians throughout the Western world are turning to bioenergetic models in growing numbers. Let us now examine the two most popular of these models—homeopathy and Chinese medicine.

Table 1: The Basic Properties of Bioenergy

Bioenergy:

1. Originates in the sun and accompanies solar rays.

2. Is contained within all living matter.

3. Has a quality of pulsation (radiation, emanation).

4. Is connected to and dependent on respiration.

5. Is affected by the weather.

6. Is affected by emotional and mental states.

7. Fluctuates over a daily cycle (twenty-four hours).

8. Behaves differently from electricity.

9. Can be conducted. (Besides metal and water, it is also conductible along glass, resin, silk and other organic substances.)

10. Can be stored in a specialized container.

11. Can affect other living matter over a distance.

12. Can be used for healing.

13. Directs the process of growth (including healing) from birth to death.

14. Can be controlled by the mind.

15. Exhibits polarity.

16. Can be communicated.

17. Can be reflected like light.

18. Flows in the direction of higher concentrations. (This is in opposition to the principle of entropy, the second law of thermodynamics. It is for this reason that bioenergy is able to establish order from disorder, thus promoting healing and regeneration.)

Table 2: Synonyms for Bioenergy or Related Phenomenon

Huang Ti	CHI	Driesch	ENTELECHY
Dashka	PRANA	Kammerer	FORMATIVE ENERGY
Pythagorus	PNEUMA	Muller	HUMAN EMOTIONS
Hippocrates	PHYSIS OR VIS MEDICTRIX	Richards	BIOMORPHS
Paracelsus	QUINTESSENCE	Burr	1) ELECTRODYNAMIC FIELDS
Helmont	ARCHEUS		2) ELECTROSTATIC FIELDS
Fludd	THE FLUID		3) QUASI ELECTRO-STATIC FIELDS
Stahl	ANIMA		4) LIFE FIELDS
Hahnemann	VITAL FORCE		5) L-FIELDS
Mesmer	ANIMAL MAGNETISM	Gurvich	MITOGENIC RADIATION
Galvani	LIFE FORCE	Reich	ORGONE ENERGY
Reichenbach	THE ODIC FORCE	Brunler	DIELECTRIC BIO-COSMIC ENERGY
Baraduc	LA FORCE VITALE	Selye	ADAPTIVE ENERGY
Kilner	THE HUMAN ATMOSPHERE (AURA)	Inyushin	BIO-PLASMA
Blondot	N-RAYS	Motoyami	KI
Barety	NEURIC ENERGY	Miller	PARAELECTRICITY
Abrams	1) PHYSICAL ENERGY 2) PSYCHIC ENERGY 3) AURIC ENERGY	Tiller	PSYCHO ENERGETIC FIELDS
Boirac	NERVE RADIOACTIVITY	Sheldrake	MORPHOGENETIC FIELDS
Bergson	ELAN VITAL	Nordestrom	BIOLOGICALLY CLOSED CIRCUITRY

3

Homeopathy:
A Bioenergetic Medicine

"It is clear that we are going out of the age of chemical and mechanical medicine and into the age of energetic and homeopathic medicine."
> William Tiller, Ph.D.,[1]
> Stanford University

"Homeopathy . . . cures a larger percentage of cases than any other method of treatment and is beyond doubt safer and more economical and the most complete medical science."
> Mahatma Gandhi[2]

Mahatma Gandhi, a leader of great vision, realized homeopathy's potential for his country—a safe, effective medicine that would be affordable for the people. In India today there are over one hundred thousand homeopathic physicians and one hundred and twenty homeopathic colleges. Homeopathy, in existence for almost two hundred years, is practiced in every industrial country in the world. In Great Britain, for example, the Royal Family has endorsed homeopathy for over one hundred years, and today Queen Elizabeth II and her family utilize a homeopathic physician. Prince Charles and other prominent Britons are promoting homeopathy, calling for a synthesis of biochemical and bioenergetical approaches which they call "complementary medicine." Complementary medicine aims to work with and amplify the innate healing power of the body, and in this way to prevent and cure disease as well as improve the overall quality of health.

Homeopathy has a long and rich tradition in Europe and

America. Almost two hundred years ago Samuel Hahnemann, a medical pioneer, emerged from Germany with a radically different system of medicine which he named homeopathy. This word derives from two Greek words, *homoios* which means "similar" and *pathos* which means "disease" or "suffering." The homeopathic pharmacological principle is referred to as "the law of similars" and is based on the observation that "like cures like." Hahnemann discovered that an overdose of any substance, plant, mineral, animal product, or chemical causes its own pattern of symptoms. He also discovered that tiny doses of this same substance could cure this specific symptom pattern. The well-known herb, *Belladonna*, is poisonous. In excessive doses the herb causes death, in moderate doses it creates hot, feverish states, and in tiny homeopathic doses it can cure certain types of fevers, flus, and inflammatory states.

Biochemical medicine, on the other hand, is based on the *allopathic* principle. *Allo* means "different from." Drugs are prescribed which produce effects that differ from those of the disease treated. These allopathic drugs tend to fight or eradicate biochemical disorders; they often bear the prefix "anti," as in the case of "antibiotics" or "antihistamine."

Through the years of rigorous experiment and trials, Hahnemann developed homeopathy into a highly sophisticated system of medicine based on bioenergy. He and his colleagues established the basic principles that guided this healing science: the recognition that the organism has inherent homeostatic self-healing capacities; the law of similars; the testing of drugs on healthy people; the strict individualization of the medicines to the person; and the use of microdoses rather than large doses.

One of Hahnemann's most important discoveries was the unique preparation of homeopathic drugs, most commonly called *remedies*. Very small doses of the remedies are utilized; these doses are prepared through a unique process of dilution and succussion (vigorous shaking). The remedies are bioenergetic, and because they work with the bioenergy of the body, amplifying the innate drive for homeostasis, they do not cause side effects. In homeopathy, disease is ultimately an energetic disharmony and can best be balanced by the appropriate stimulus, the microdose. We therefore call homeopathy a "bioenergetical medical science." It is, as we shall explain, both thorough and complex in its theory and practice.

During the nineteenth century, homeopathy spread through Europe, gaining a small but enthusiastic following. Along the way it met much resistance from conventional doctors, but because of the success of homeopathic treatments—for example, in the terrible epidemics of the time—homeopathy soon spread to other parts of the world. Homeopathy flourished in nineteenth century America attracting such notable admirers as Mark Twain, William James, and John D. Rockefeller Sr.[3] At the turn of the century, about 15 percent of American doctors used homeopathic remedies, but with the discovery of "miracle" drugs, such as insulin and penicillin, homeopathy soon appeared outdated and unscientific. Subsequently, advocates of homeopathy lost political battles with the allopathic doctors and the number of homeopathic physicians dwindled significantly. Many allopathic doctors considered homeopathy a system based on placebo response.

Today, the situation has not changed much. The use of microdoses and the concept of bioenergy are ideas not readily acceptable to the current mechanistic model. Recently, however, there has been a subtle shift in the attitude toward homeopathic treatment. Conventional science is beginning to examine holistic concepts in areas such as quantum physics, and presently we are seeing signs of a more open attitude towards homeopathy. The prestigious British medical journal, *The Lancet*, recently published a favorable clinical trial of homeopathy. This and other recent studies published in respected journals point to a new direction in medicine. Homeopathic principles, once seen as implausible, are being examined in a new light. It is not an exaggeration to say that homeopathy is now experiencing a renaissance, especially when one considers the new interest in bioenergetic phenomena and research.

Study of the theories of homeopathy reveals a surprising wealth of knowledge, some of it pertinent to the very frontiers of modern science: quantum physics, gestalt psychology, and the systems theory of biology. Homeopathy requires a broad vision. One cannot approach it from the narrow perspective of the specialist, because it demands an intelligence capable of spanning and integrating different ideas and experiences, and combining left- and right-brain thinking.

Health and Homeostasis

One of the fulcrums upon which bioenergetic medicine rests is the phenomenon of homeostasis. In biochemical medicine there is no clear definition of health; in fact, it is often defined in negation, as "the absence of disease and pain." In Chinese medicine and homeopathy, a clear vision of health is the foundation of theory and practice. Homeostasis, specifically the equilibrium of bioenergy, is one of the foundations of homeopathy and offers clues to the action and efficacy of homeopathic practice.

In the bioenergetic model, the body is pictured as an integrated system which has an innate drive for balance and health. In the biochemical model disease is often seen as an invasion from outside, hostile forces, but from the bioenergetic point of view, the picture is more complex. In many cases, disease is a sign that the body is striving to maintain balance, to adjust, and to adapt. Hans Selye gives the simple example of the inflammation around a splinter; the inflammatory process is a result of protective mechanisms. Symptoms often seen as negative can be signs of the body adapting to new stress factors. This idea is being recognized in conventional medicine. The common response to a fever, for example, is to give aspirin to lower the temperature; fevers, however, can rid the body of unwanted bacteria and other toxins. Rather than suppressing a fever with drugs, homeopaths will work *with* the body by speeding the healing response with a suitable remedy.

The concept of homeostasis has existed for centuries in systems like Chinese medicine and homeopathy, but it has yet to be integrated into allopathic practice. William Cannon, one of the first modern doctors to examine homeostasis, wrote the classic, *The*

Wisdom of the Body. This work, published in the 1930s, was not enthusiastically accepted by his colleagues because it was ahead of its time. Cannon studied the multiplicity of homeostatic systems of the body, such as breathing, temperature control and blood pressure, and established that they were controlled by a complex feedback mechanism. He went far in his research, even recognizing the effect of mental stress on physical functions, but he never envisioned a fundamental unity in the body. He did observe, however, that distressing symptoms, rather than being disease factors, were often signals of the body adapting to stress. This last idea was developed by his student, Hans Selye, who is now world reknowned for his research into stress and health.

Dr. Selye has made a lifelong study of the effects of stress on the body. He demonstrated with countless experiments that the body has a generalized response to stress factors—heat, cold, trauma, shock, bacteria, etc.—and that when the body is continuously threatened, the overall homeostasis is upset. The body responds to the myriad stress factors with what Selye called "adaptive energy." He explains:

> Many diseases are not actually so much the direct result of some external agent (an infection or intoxication) as they are the consequence of the body's inability to meet these agents with adequate adaptive reactions, . . .[4]

Selye is not alone in his research; many other scientists have come to similar conclusions. Ludwig von Bertalanffy, one of the founders of the general systems theory, has emphasized the importance of homeostasis to the body. Systems theory states that every living organism follows an inherent law of life by striving to maintain balance. The aim of the organism is to achieve a steady state, a relative homeostasis of functions, by adjusting and adopting to the myriad stress factors of life.

It is of special interest that Selye, after decades of research, came to the conclusion that the body has some unknown form of energy that balances these stress factors. He states:

It is as though something were lost, or used up, during the work of adaptation; but what this is we do not know. The term adaptation energy has been coined for that which is consumed during the continued adaptive work to indicate that it is something different from the caloric energy we receive from our food, but this is only a name, and even now—almost thirty years after this hypothesis was first formulated—we still have no precise concept of what this energy might be. Further research along these lines would seem to hold great promise, since here we appear to touch upon the fundamental fact of fatigue and aging.[5]

This resonant quote, from one of the premier medical researchers of this century, gives the impression that Selye was close to resurrecting the concept of bioenergy. What he proposes is really one of the great medical challenges, perhaps more valuable than the development of artificial organs: How can we prevent the degeneration of organs in the first place?

One can see the progression from Cannon on homeostasis, to Selye on adaptive energy and stress factors, to the present day when medical researchers are examining the body/mind connection. "Adaptive energy," or "healing response," is the work the body/mind does to reestablish balance. That work involves more than one specialized area; it entails the whole body—the brain, the nervous system, the endocrine glands, the immune system, and organ systems—working together as a unit. This holistic model is thus difficult to verify by conventional methods which require the isolation and observation of a particular organ or system. Nonetheless, current research is beginning to examine facets of this healing response, and recently there has been a surge of interest in the relationship of the brain to the immune system. The effect of thoughts and emotions on the disease process is a phenomenon that can no longer be ignored. In fact, this connection is now being studied by scientists around the world. Recent studies at Harvard have demonstrated that stressful emotions such as prolonged grief can compromise the immune system.[6] This interface of the immune system and the brain is an exciting new field that promises to reveal many biochemical facts about the body/mind connection, and to open the way for a greater acceptance of holistic theory.

Homeopathy is a unique Western medical system because of its bioenergetic focus. Each homeopathic remedy is a specific picture of a bioenergetic pattern of disharmony that includes physical, emotional, and mental symptoms. Because like cures like, the remedy must match the totality of the patient's condition and in this way stimulate the homeostasis of body/mind. To explain how homeopathic treatment works, we like to use the analogy of the harmonic resonance that can occur between two tones of music. Because of sympathetic vibration the tones amplify each other. The body vibrates at certain frequencies in health, but in disease these vibrations become weak, static, or irregular. Remedies of similar vibrational frequencies stimulate the healing by balancing and regulating the bioenergetic system. With this principle in mind we will now examine the law of similars, the very heart of homeopathy.

The Law of Similars

The law of similars can be found in many ancient and modern medical systems. It wasn't until the nineteenth century, however, that the law of similars became the core of a complete system of medicine, mainly through the efforts of Samuel Hahnemann. He was a medical doctor and researcher, as well as one of the foremost experts of his day in chemistry and pharmacology.[7] A brilliant intellectual, Hahnemann could read French, Hebrew, Greek, Latin, English, and German, and was therefore able to study many of the classic works of medical history. From all these sources he acquired a phenomenal knowledge of pharmacology, which he used to develop the remarkable homeopathic pharmaceopoeia.

Through Hahnemann's strenuous efforts—including years of self-experimentation—and his insistence upon meticulous observation, homeopathy developed into a sophisticated medical science. Like Chinese medicine, homeopathy is a pragmatic system of healing that respects the underlying intelligence of nature, and extracts its principles from a careful observation of sick and healthy people.

Hahnemann, an exacting scientist, once said:

> Homeopathy appeals solely to the verdict of experience . . .
> Repeat the experiment, carefully and accurately, and you will
> find the doctrine confirmed at every step . . . Homeopathy insists
> on being judged by its results.[8]

Hahnemann's discontent with the medicine of his day led him
on a quest for a new model of therapeutics. Throughout his research and translations of medical texts, he was looking for clues
to the principles of healing. In 1796 his own children became sick,
which pressured him to intensify his search for a safe, effective,
and scientific form of medicine. During that pivotal year he became inspired to perform an experiment on himself. This experiment was his great turning point, opening up a vast new world
of medicine previously hidden to man. From this fortunate act
he went on to develop the science of homeopathy.

While translating Cullen's *Materia Medica* into German,
he became intrigued by Cullen's lengthy discussion of "Peruvian
Bark." Peruvian Bark, the source of quinine, was used to treat
malaria. Cullen claimed it was effective because of its tonic properties to the stomach and its bitter astringent qualities. Hahnemann
questioned this assumption. Rather than avoiding the question,
he became inspired to test Cullen's hypothesis. He decided to try
the drug on himself—a bold act, for that or any other time, as
few doctors have tested drugs on themselves (preferring to use their
patients or animals instead).

In this now famous quote he recalled:

> I took for several days, as an experiment, four drams of good
> China (Peruvian Bark) twice daily. My feet, finger tips, etc.,
> at first became cold; I became languid and drowsy; then my
> heart began to palpitate; my pulse became quick and hard; and
> intolerable anxiety and trembling (but without rigor); prostra-
> tion in all the limbs; then pulsation in the head, redness of the
> cheeks, thirst; briefly all the symptoms associated with intermit-
> tent fever in succession. . . . I discontinued the medicine, and
> I was once more in good health.[9]

Hahnemann experienced the basic symptoms of malaria. He

had discovered that Peruvian Bark created symptoms similar to malaria, and thus deduced that it worked because of the law of similars. Subsequently, all homeopathic remedies have been subjected to such tests, called "provings." These provings are always performed on healthy volunteers, and the range of symptoms that each substance produces indicates its curative potential. With this inspired experiment, one of the hidden masterpieces of medical history, Hahnemann opened a door to a new world of clinical medicine based on the law of similars. The law of similars is deceptively simple and requires much thought and experience to understand fully.

In his major book, the *Organon of Medicine,* an underground classic of medical history, Hahnemann states: "A drug produces an artificial disease. Like any other foreign material, it provides a specific stimulus. Its only curative effect lies in eliciting a reaction from the organism."[10] A drug that in large doses can cause unpleasant symptoms, can, in small doses, cure those very symptoms. This is a principle of pharmacological drug action that applies best to homeopathic microdoses. The remedies, as we shall soon describe in more detail, are highly diluted, and it is best to use these tiny doses to activate the healing response. Larger doses can be harmful. Since the remedy is harmonic in action and the dose minute, toxicity, so common with chemical drugs, does not occur. The verification of this law, simple to reproduce, is unknown or unaccepted by regular medicine. The common attitude is that "it can't possibly work, so why test it?"

The ancient Chinese, aware of the law of similars, refer to it in the *Nei Ching,* one of their medical texts.[11] The ancient Greeks also discuss this principle; indeed, the famous physician, Hippocrates, taught that "through the similar disease developing and through the employment of the similar, the disease is healed."[12] And it is not surprising that Paracelsus, the Swiss doctor and alchemist of the sixteenth century, wrote about and applied this healing principle.[13] In the annals of folk medicine, one can find references and examples of "like cures like." American Indians, for example, employed 'hot' herbs like cayenne for fevers, and prescribed a medicine made from bee venom for swollen joints—an application verified by modern medicine and homeopathy. In the modern age there are many examples of applications of the law of similars: allergy shots, vaccines, and radiation for cancer (radiation can cause cancer). However, these examples are not true homeopathy because they do not individualize each case and do not use the specially-prepared microdoses.

It is interesting to observe how many of the modern drugs work because of the laws of similars. At least three of these drugs (digitalis, nitroglycerine, and gold) were prescribed by homeopaths before their acceptance into modern practice. Even more significantly, modern pharmacology has not yet fully explained how these drugs work. Homeopaths, however, affirm that they work because they can cause the symptoms that they cure.

Homeopathic Drug Provings

Hahnemann's discovery of the law of similars was an experiment that revealed a vast new world of medical therapeutics. The key to this world is the drug trials called "provings." A proving is conducted on a group of healthy volunteers. The homeopathic remedy is given daily in crude or potentized doses to the volunteers until subjective and objective symptoms are obtained. Any changes in the volunteers are carefully observed and noted. Symptoms that emerge can be as diverse as any experienced by sick people, ranging from common physical symptoms such as a throbbing pain in the right temple, to more complex mental symptoms such as a tendency to forget certain words while speaking. The specific characteristics of each symptom, whether objective or subjective, is extremely important and noted meticulously by the subject and experimenter.

This kind of testing is very different from drug trials with animals; these allopathic experiments only study the pathological aspects of disease. Homeopathic testing uses healthy *people* as the measure of drug characteristics, thus revealing the full dimensional picture of these remedies. It is interesting how so many homeopathic principles seem diametrically opposed to allopathic practice. Their completely different approach to drug testing is yet another example of this dynamic polarity. However, it is important to emphasize that homeopathic doctors fully recognize the value of biochemical drug testing.

Because homeopathic remedies induce what is called an "artificial disease," the symptoms that emerge from a proving disappear soon after its use is terminated. The provings are not dangerous or unhealthy because the microdose remedies simply mimic different symptoms of illness. In fact, Hahnemann himself—who participated in over ninety provings—lived a long, robust life of eighty-nine years.

In time, the key symptoms gathered from each proving will enter the homeopathic *materia medica,* the reference book for the remedies. In the *materica medica,* several pages are devoted to each major remedy, displaying the full range of physical, emotional, and mental symptoms. Some remedies are relatively simple, relating to a specific organ or acute symptom profile; others are highly complex, encompassing the totality of life functions. In Chapter Seven we will describe fourteen homeopathic remedy pictures, demonstrating their detail and depth.

Provings of homeopathic remedies have been retested and verified by doctors since Hahnemann's time, a testament to his capabilities.[14] Besides the provings, other information about remedies has come from clinical experience and reports of drug poisoning. When a person ingests a poisonous plant, he or she inadvertently does a crude proving. A simple example would be smoking a cigarette. To people not accustomed to tobacco, it often produces an unpleasant queasiness and lightheadedness, symptoms that homeopathic tobacco can cure. Homeopathic tobacco, for example, can be prescribed to alleviate the symptoms of motion sickness (since it creates, in overdose, similar symptoms).

Homeopathic Casetaking and Prescribing

What is so unique and significant about homeopathic casetaking is the careful individualization of the total range of symptoms. In provings, for example, the homeopathic remedy *Pulsatilla* (the windflower) produces a vivid picture of physical and psychological characteristics. The typical *Pulsatilla* patients are marked by their emotional temperament; they are gentle, mild, and moody, with a yearning for attention and tendency to weep. Chief physical symptoms include wandering pains, symptoms that change frequently, a lack of thirst, symptoms aggravated by heat, and secretions of thick, bland mucus. They feel better when consoled and when out of doors, and their symptoms can be aggravated by hot, stuffy rooms. They are prone to digestive problems and cannot tolerate fatty food. The remedy is effective for a variety of conditions, like hay fevers, colds and menstrual problems, but only if the patient displays the major characteristics of *Pulsatilla*.

Even in this simplified picture of a remedy, one can envision the multidimensional emphases of homeopathic casetaking. Without too much prodding or directing, the physician has to elicit a complex range of symptoms from the patient, and then he must determine the best remedy.

A patient might come into the clinic complaining of sinus problems. He presents a complex array of symptoms, some of which clearly indicate *Pulsatilla*, some of which do not. The doctor must then differentiate between *Pulsatilla* and other similar remedies. Once he has chosen the most similar remedy, the *simillimum*, he will then prescribe several doses to the patient and ask him to return for a follow-up. The homeopath will not give excessive repetitions of the remedy because the microdose, in just the right quantity, is sufficient to stimulate a healing response.

Though there is a system of prescribing mixed remedies, the classical homeopath, following in the footsteps of Hahnemann, matches the person with one remedy (which in time can change). The reasoning behind this important principle lies in the nature of the provings: one remedy is proved at a time. A remedy represents a wave form that must correspond in totality to the patient's energetic pattern. Several remedies can confuse the energetic response, creating interfering patterns. This contradiction, however, does not invalidate prescribing mixed remedies because they too have a pattern, even though this has not been depicted in provings. Incidently, the incorrect homeopathic remedy will for the most part do nothing—there is no resonance, therefore no response.

Homeopathic casetaking and prescribing are complex subjects that we will return to in a later chapter.

Hering's Law

Dr. Constantine Hering, one of Hahnemann's most famous students, migrated to America and became one of the great American homeopaths. He was a founder of Hahnemann Medical College in Philadelphia and author of several important homeopathic texts. Hering added one more cornerstone to homeopathic theory, now called Hering's Law. This principle, of great importance in homeopathy, is found in other systems of natural medicine but generally not so developed. Hering's Law points to a special property of bioenergetic healing.

When the bioenergy of the body is properly stimulated by the right stimulus (a microdose, for example), the patient might feel temporarily worse. This brief aggravation is the nature of the healing (or adaptive) process. Healing involves change; in the process of restoring balance, changes occur in the bioenergy and physical functions, creating transient discomfort, which soon results in better overall health and wellbeing.

A patient comes into the clinic complaining of migraines that return every two or three weeks. After taking the correct remedy, the same migraine reoccurs, an aggravation that is followed quickly by amelioration. The person feels much better and finds that the headaches steadily diminish. The aggravation is a clear indication that the remedy worked. It does not always occur, but when it does, it clearly indicates a curative response.

Hering's Law is the culmination of years of clinical observation of thousands of patients. Hering noted that the healing aggravation often follows a particular pattern (a fact most useful in the clinic). The order of this pattern is that symptoms, in general, disappear "from within outward, from above downward, from the more important to the less important organs, and in reverse order of appearance." Homeopaths recognize a hierarchy of symptoms. For example, mental or emotional symptoms are more important in casetaking than physical ones; symptoms of the head and torso are more important than those of lesser organs. Also noted is the curious phenomenon that symptoms reappear in reverse order of their appearance, a phenomenon we see in the following case: A patient comes in complaining of asthma. After being prescribed the appropriate remedy, he experiences a temporary reoccurence of eczema, from which he suffered two years previously. It turns out that the eczema was treated by cortisone which suppressed the problem and pushed it into deeper levels of the body, resulting in asthma. The correct remedy, by triggering homeostasis, releases the previous suppression from the deeper levels, effecting a discharge to the surface which is then followed by better health. Hering's Law is important because it displays the path of natural healing following the appropriate bioenergetic stimulus.

The Microdose Enigma

After his famous Peruvian Bark experiment, Hahnemann made another great discovery. He began to reduce the quantity of the drugs and found that smaller doses worked more efficiently and safely. At the same time he was inspired to try something new. With each serial dilution of the remedy, he shook the vial; by repeatedly and forcibly pounding the liquid-filled vial, Hahnemann found that he could enhance the therapeutic action of the remedy as well as reducing its toxic effect.

One of the paradoxes of homeopathy is that specially-prepared minute doses are more therapeutic than crude doses. When working with bioenergy, subtle action is the most effective therapy. The microdoses can best catalyze the adaptive processes, facilitated by the action of the law of similars. In homeopathy, the adage "less is more" is especially apt.

In Hahnemann's time, people were not even vaguely familiar

with the microscopic world of bacteria, viruses, or with the power of minute chemicals like hormones. Therefore the concept of microdoses was considered preposterous. Hahnemann, undeterred, saw the dramatic clinical action of these tiny doses. In fact, he utilized a little-known pharmacological principle of modern times, now called the Arndt-Shultz Law, which recognizes the biphasic action of drugs: large and small doses have an opposite effect. Every drug has a stimulating effect in small doses, while larger doses inhibit, and much larger ones kill.[15] Modern medicine has yet to explore the subtle applications of this principle.

It is important to emphasize that there are two actions necessary to prepare a homeopathic remedy: dilution and succussion. As an example, we will explain the preparation of an herb, *Gelsemium* (yellow jasmine), a common homeopathic remedy. The mother tincture is prepared from the root of the plant according to strict pharmacological standards. One drop of the tincture is then mixed with nine drops of distilled water (or pure alcohol). This dilution is then *succussed* (forcibly shaken), adding kinetic energy to the mixture and releasing the therapeutic essence of the plant. This results in a 1x dilution, the "x" signifying the decimal or one in ten dilutions. One drop of this 1x dilution is then removed, placed in a sterile vial, and nine drops of the water are added, followed again by a succussion. This process of dilution and succussion is then repeated four more times, resulting in a 6x remedy. Another preparation, centessimal or "c," is also used, the dilutions made on a scale of one to a hundred rather than one to ten. These liquid remedies can then be applied to tiny lactose pellets which will be stored in glass vials, ready for use. This procedure of making a remedy must be followed with utmost care to ensure the purity and effectiveness of the final product. Modern homeopathic pharmacies offer the best in new techniques and sterile conditions.

The action of dilution and succussion produces a "potentized" homeopathic remedy, a medicine that works bioenergetically. The remedies are used in varying potencies. Sometimes homeopaths will use mother tinctures or allopathic drugs, but more often he uses remedies that range from low to medium to high potency. A 6x or 6c would be a low potency, a 30c or 60x would be a medium potency, and a 200c or 1000x would be a high potency. Paradoxically, the more dilute solutions are considered more potent. The rate of vibration of the remedy is raised exponentially with repeated dilution and succussion.

As science has penetrated into the microscopic world over the past hundred years, it has become increasingly apparent that microdoses have a profound effect on all levels of life. A good example is the incredible power locked in atoms, power so great that it can cause a chain reaction of mass destruction. In biology and physiology there are countless examples of the power of minute chemical doses. The human body, for example, depends on the action of minute amounts of hormones. One recently-discovered hormone exists in one part per trillion in the blood;[16] in time, others occurring in even more minute amounts will be found.

In 1981, an interesting scientific paper was published by a British biologist, A.R. Stebbing.[17] From scientific studies around the world, he has compiled data supporting the potency of microdoses. Stebbing uses the term "hormesis" to describe the physiological activity of minute doses. The concept of hormesis is a modern version of the previously-mentioned Arndt-Shultz principle: large doses can inhibit or kill; small doses can stimulate. For example, it is known that large doses of antibiotics can kill (a useful fact in medicine), while smaller doses can actually increase the growth of animals, fungi, and protozoa.[18] Stebbing suggests that hormesis is a far more common occurrence in nature than is accepted, and that there is resistance to studying this phenomenon because its action is unknown. No doubt the law of similars is a clue to this mystery.

The above examples validate the action of minute doses, but only among the lower potencies (up to 6x or 10x). Potencies beyond 12c or 30x exceed the limit where any molecules would be present, an absurd proposition by conventional standards. These figures exceed Avogadro's number (10^{-23}), a limit in chemistry beyond which no molecules would exist. Therefore, we are examining two kinds of microdoses: those that contain measurable molecules and those that do not. Are these higher-potency remedies placebos? Or are we dealing with a phenomenon that exceeds the present theoretical boundaries of chemistry and physics? Ironically, it has been clinically demonstrated by several generations of homeopaths that these higher potencies are not only effective; they are more potent than the lower doses!

An ultra-modern measuring technique, nuclear magnetic resonance spectroscopy, studies the spin of protons in a molecule. This technique has been applied to the study of high-potency homeopathic remedies with positive results.[19] Two researchers, Barnard and Stephenson, hypothesized that what is important in these high-potency dilutions is not the chemicals of the solute (the substance being diluted) but the overall structure of the solvent (the water in which the substance is being diluted).[20] Possibly the action of dilution and succussion induces an electromagnetic patterning of the water. The original substance, once potentized, releases a template—a preatomic dynamic patterning—into the water. We call these remedies "bioenergetic patterns," a specific configuration that influences the bioenergy.

Though the workings of homeopathy might seem mysterious, the efficacy of the medicine is evident. Decades of experience with severely sick people and animals confirms its effectiveness, as does experimental work with animals, plants, yeast, and bacteria. Furthermore, it has been demonstrated that homeopathic remedies have measurable effects on living organisms. Therefore, we should not be apprehensive about these presently unexplained elements of homeopathy. Science is full of unproven theories, and some of our basic facts of life, such as gravity or the mechanism of hormones, have yet to be fully explained. Homeopathy involves a level of physics and biology that is just now being revealed by sophisticated new methods and technology. A hundred years ago, after all, x-rays were a complete mystery.

It is easy to judge or criticize homeopathy from a biochemical point of view. From the perspective of this model, homeopathy seems highly dubious. However, it cannot be passed over so readily because it involves multi-dimensional perspectives of man and health. The biochemical model can be pictured as a straight line, while homeopathy is a circle. Explaining homeopathy to a linear person is like Columbus trying to explain to his contemporaries that the earth is round. Biochemical medicine is based on a linear perspective of chemicals, biochemical change, and pathology, and while this approach is valid, it only looks at part of the picture.

Homeopathy, like Chinese medicine, infers that there is some formative intelligence in the universe. Modern medicine, a product of a mechanistic era, does not acknowledge such an underlying sentient influence. This profound philosophical divergence has generated completely different perspectives of health and disease. The essential mystery of homeopathy may not be explained away simply by biochemical interactions; the mystery of homeopathy is the mystery of life. Erwin Chargraff, the biochemist who discovered the pairing of DNA and thus opened the way for the understanding of gene structure, expresses this enigma when he wrote of biology, "No other science deals in its very name with a subject that it cannot define."

Homeopathy and Scientific Validation

The purpose of this section is not to provide a complete picture of homeopathic scientific research, but we would like to offer the reader a glimpse into this crucial topic. At this point, it is important to emphasize that homeopathy does not in any way divorce itself from conventional medicine. The true genius of homeopathy is that it has expanded the scope of conventional medicine to include holistic principles based on the sound principles of verification and testing. Homeopathy is a rigorous art and science that takes years to master and includes conventional training in biochemical medicine. Homeopaths are not dogmatically opposed to surgery when it is required, nor do they oppose the use of allopathic drugs in certain instances.

Besides almost 200 years of clinical validation, homeopathy

has also been tested in the laboratory. More work is needed to convince the skeptics, but each year new scientific support for homeopathy emerges. Currently, homeopathic research is rarely funded by government grants or university subsidies, and homeopaths have been forced to progress on their own meager financial resources. Nonetheless, there are many examples of excellent research.

For several decades, W. Boyd, a Scottish scientist, performed exacting laboratory experiments using homeopathic remedies.[21] One example is his study of the effect of homeopathic mercurious chloride (H_3Cl_2) in varying potencies on the activity of diastase, an enzyme. These potencies were demonstrated to stimulate the hydrolysis of starch above the water controls. Boyd's research was impeccable in all details and has been supported by statistical analysis. Other scientists (Krause and others, 1981) have also worked with homeopathic remedies and demonstrated their effect on enzyme activity.[22]

Another kind of homeopathic testing comes from the progressive Boiron Laboratories in France.[23] They have conducted many experiments on the action of homeopathic doses. One involved radioactive tracers to study the effect of homeopathic arsenic on the accumulation and elimination of arsenic from poisoned rats. The results indicate that *Arsenic 7c* does indeed speed up the elimination of toxic doses of arsenic. Similar experiments have been performed using other poisons. This kind of experimentation clearly indicates that homeopathy has another value in this era of chemical pollutants.

From another field completely unconnected to homeopathy is an ingenious experiment published in *Science* (1977), involving the spraying of agricultural crops with diluted fertilizers.[24] Faced with the threat of dwindling petrochemical fertilizers, Dr. Stanley Ries and his colleagues decided to search for a less expensive alternative. They extracted an alcohol from alfalfa, a very nutritious crop, and diluted this mixture to 10^{-9}, what would approximately equal a 9x homeopathic dose. They did not succuss these dilutions. After spraying this extremely minute dose on crops, they found a substantial difference between these and the control group and unsprayed crops. Yields in a variety of crops sprayed with the dilutions were 20–60% higher.

Because of inadequate finances and other obstacles, there have not been many clinical trials of homeopathy that meet the standards of biochemical testing. However, this pattern is changing; in the past five years, the results of a few homeopathic trials have appeared in regular medical journals. This is a great advance for homeopathy as it indicates that the walls of automatic resistance are gradually breaking down. One test appeared in the *British Journal of Clinical Pharmacology* (1980) involving a double-blind trial of rheumatoid arthritis, which shows an 82% improvement for those given individually chosen remedies, as opposed to only 21% for those given placebos.[25]

Another trial, appearing in *The Lancet*, the prestigious British medical journal, involved hay fever patients and demonstrated that the homeopathic remedies were effective. This study was a unique colloboration between homeopathic and allopathic doctors at a hospital in Scotland.[26]

A well-controlled trial was conducted during World War II in London and Glasgow where different homeopathic remedies were used in the prevention and treatment of mustard gas burns (Patterson, 1944).[27] A reanalysis of the data using current statistical methods demonstrated the value of homeopathic therapy.

As an aside, it is sad to notice how little homeopathic research has come out of America as compared to India, France, Germany, and England, where there are more medical alternatives. This trend, however, is changing as Americans turn to homeopathy in increasing numbers. A sign of positive change is the recent establishment of the Foundation For Homeopathic Education and Research. More information about research and homeopathy can be found in Dana Ullman's *Homeopathy: Medicine for the 21st Century* and in Harris Coulter's *Homeopathic Science and Modern Medicine.*

New Directions:
How Do Homeopathic Remedies
Interface with the Body?

The potentials of homeopathic research are fascinating because they involve the mysteries of life and health. In this section we will examine a new line of thinking regarding the action of homeopathic microdoses.

As incredible as it might seem, H_2O—the common water molecule—is implicated in unravelling these questions. Water is a remarkable substance. It is the universal solvent, the fundamental medium of all living things, and it is absolutely essential for all life. Even though H_2O seems simple, it is very complex and has unique properties which contain some of the secrets of health and life. The body, after all, is about 70% water; the brain, 90%; the blood, 98%. What is especially interesting is that this omnipresent and supposedly simple molecule is still somewhat a mystery. In fact, no scientist to date has fully revealed the structural secrets of water.[28]

Of related importance is the underlying crystalline structure of all living things (such as bone, protein, and DNA). The crystal matrix, best exemplified in the quartz crystal (the basis of computer chips), is a universal pattern fundamental to the order of life—the seed of many forms of organic and inorganic life.[29] This crystal configuration holds a key, not yet fully understood, to the underlying patterns of life, and is closely connected to the overall structure and arrangment of water molecules. How do individual water molecules relate to each other? Is there an overall pattern that governs these water molecules, particularly in living organisms?

The particular arrangment and interrelation of water molecules is an intriguing question, one that has far-ranging implications for health and life. Water molecules are found in different patterns in nature: snow, fog, clouds, ice, liquid. Generally, it is assumed that in the liquid form the individual molecules are arranged *randomly*. There is, however, growing evidence that these water molecules are structured, forming semi-crystalline patterns held together by bioenergetic forces.[30]

P.W. Bridgeman, former chairman of the Harvard department of physics, researched the effects of freezing water at different altitudes.[31] He found that at high altitudes a particular ice crystallization pattern was formed, different from those of lower altitudes. Of special interest is that when melted ice from the higher altitude is refrozen at lower altitudes, it maintains the pattern of the higher altitude. This clearly suggests that the structuring of water can be imprinted without adding any new substance to the water.

Since our bodies are primarily water, it is no surprise that the crystalline structuring of water could have profound effect on our health. Fluids bathe all tissues and cells of the body; blood is the fluid nourishment of the cells, and all chemical activities take place in a fluid environment. All the life processes of the body depend on water.

How can water become structured? It is suggested that this structuring is influenced by bioenergy. Regular tap water is unstructured. It has little or no underlying dynamic pattern, but once influenced by *living* energy, such as the sun, it becomes structured.[32] The water molecules arrange themselves in a dynamic semi-crystalline pattern which allows for further attraction to the life energy. If this is true, then the healthy, robust body would have a predominance of structured fluids which enhances all physiological activities. In disease these patterns are weak or irregular which, quite obviously, diminishes health and well-being, and leads in time to degenerative diseases like cancer.

Hypothetically, homeopathic remedies work because of the underlying patterning of water. As has been suggested, the potentizing of a remedy influences the dynamic pattern of the solvent (the water in which the substance is potentized). The original substance from which the remedy is made restructures the water through the process of dilution and succussion. Succussion, so crucial to homeopathic pharmacology, creates a collision between molecules which quantitizes them and increases their rate of vibration.[33] Dr. Paul Callinan, an Australian physicist, recently presented an impressive theoretical analysis of the microdose phenomenon to his country's parliament. He hypothesizes that succussion and dilution produce energy storage in the bonds of the dilution in the infrared spectrum which "downloads" in contact with water in living systems.[34] This simply means that there is an energy transfer from the potentized water to the fluids of the body. The potentized remedy, of a specific energetic configuration, influences the water like liquid crystal and restructures the body's water which then modifies receptor sites or enzyme action.[35] This in turn triggers a process of biochemical change towards homeostasis throughout the body/mind.

These theories, however speculative, are important and stimulating for those interested in the underlying patterns of health, life, and bioenergetic medicines. Most likely, the bioelectric properties of life interface with the structuring of water, providing one of the formative influences of life. We hope that scientists and health professionals continue to explore these frontiers.

Homeopathy in the Modern World

Today, homeopathy is practised all over the world. With the expanding interest in natural medicines, homeopathy is answering a great need in the modern world. And with the increasing awareness and concern about chemical pollution of our inner and outer environment, people are eager for medicines that do not add to these problems. Since homeopathy works with the body by enhancing its innate drive for homeostasis, there is little chance of toxic side effects.

Homeopathy is used quite extensively in Europe, India, Pakistan, Mexico, and South America. In most European cities, including Moscow, one can find homeopathic physicians, clinics, and even hospitals. The Royal Homeopathic Hospital in London has existed for over one hundred years and to this day its doors are open to the public. In France an estimated 25% of the population have utilized homeopathy, and one can purchase the remedies in more than 20,000 pharmacies. In Germany there is a sizable group of doctors who are trained in homeopathy, and the German fascination for precision has inspired sophisticated electronic devices that can be used for acupuncture and homeopathy.

In the United States the situation is quite different. The AMA and pharmaceutical companies have a vested interest in not researching or supporting homeopathy. Not only is homeopathy a taboo bioenergetic medicine, it is also far more economical and hence less profitable. Despite formidable barriers, homeopathy is nevertheless resurging in this country, indicative of its practical success and of the public need. In general people are becoming more aware of the need for natural, non-toxic medicines in this age of chemical and electromagnetic pollution.

In Brazil and Argentina there are several thousand homeopathic medical doctors. The Brazilian government has sanctioned homeopathy, and it is now taught at a few medical schools. Esteemed doctors, like Dr. Fransisco Eizayaga of Argentina, teach homeopathy to hundreds of South American physicians. Dr. Eizayaga, a urologist by training, has over thirty-five years of clinical experience and is one of a new breed of modern homeopaths. With a solid foundation in pathology and homeopathy, he blends the best of both worlds without compromising the essence of classical homeopathic prescribing. Only with this quality of knowledge and experience will conventional doctors turn their heads and examine homeopathy with an open mind. And then they will see its clinical validity and value.

The core of homeopathy, however, has not changed much since Hahnemann's time because homeopathy is based on principles derived from natural laws. New remedies are discovered and used, but they do not supplant the recognized ones. Despite new technologies and knowledge, the modern homeopath still respects the skill and wisdom of the great homeopaths of the last century.

The face of homeopathy, however, is undergoing extensive changes. Computers are now employed to facilitate the selection of the right remedy. Advanced research techniques study the inner workings of homeopathy. New remedies are introduced to meet the challenges of modern health problems, such as the recent increase in immune deficiency diseases. Even new diagnostic techniques utilizing sophisticated technology are being introduced by modern homeopaths, but these we will discuss in a later chapter. From around the world many new books and studies are appearing, strongly indicative of the growing attraction to this gentle healing art. In the next two chapters we will explore the vast world of Chinese medicine, in many ways an Oriental counterpart to homeopathy—a medicine based on the phenomenon of bioenergy.

4

Introducing
Chinese Medicine

"Doctors of Western medicine and doctors of traditional
Chinese medicine have much to learn by comparing practices and by testing one another. It is time for an exchange
of medical information and positive criticism. Condescen-
sion and bias need to be unlearned and replaced with
mutual cooperation and intensive investigation."
David Eisenberg, M.D.[1]

To the average American, it seems incredible that this
ancient healing art from the Orient could have any validity in the
context of today's high-tech medical science. To the uninitiated,
the basic concepts of Chinese medicine appear to be medieval
nonsense. What with lasers, CAT scans, nuclear resonate devices
and the like, how could *yin* and *yang* ever hope to compete?
Chinese medicine, however, is a powerful approach to healing
that does not rely on conventional biochemical data. In this chapter
we will explain as simply as possible the essence of this medicine
and how it works.

Oriental medicine represents a vast body of knowledge, the
accumulation of observations made for over 5,000 years by millions
of doctors on billions of people. The first major book about this
medicine, the *Nei Ching (Inner Classics)*, was written over 2,000
years ago; it is still required reading for the Chinese doctor of
today. This book is a dialogue between Huang-Ti (The Yellow
Emperor) and his court physician, Chi Po. At the beginning of
the *Nei Ching*, the Yellow Emperor asks Chi Po why people do
not live to be one hundred and twenty like they did in ancient

times. To this Chi Po replies:

> The ancient people who knew the proper way to live had
> followed the pattern of *yin* and *yang* which is the regular pat-
> tern of heaven and earth, remained in harmony with numerical
> symbols which are the great principles of human life, eaten and
> drunken with moderation, lived their daily lives in a regular pat-
> tern with neither excess nor abuse. For this reason, their spirits
> and bodies had remained in perfect harmony with each other,
> and consequently, they could live out their natural life span and
> die at the age of over one hundred and twenty years.
>
> On the other hand, people nowadays are quite different,
> because they intoxicate themselves exorbitantly, replace a nor-
> mal life with a life of abuse, have sexual intercourse while in-
> toxicated, exhaust their pure energy though gratification of their
> desires, waste their true energy through careless and prolonged
> consumption, fail to retain their energy in abundance and to
> guard their spirits constantly, rush to the gratification of their
> hearts to the contrary of the true happiness of life, live their daily
> lives in an irregular pattern. It is for this reason that they can
> only live half of their life span.[2]

Chinese medicine is much larger in scope than the present
Western use of acupuncture suggests. Acupuncture is one branch
of Chinese medicine's eight branches which include a broad range
of theraeutics: herbs, diet, massage, manipulations, bone-setting,
exercises, and meditation. This ancient healing art is based on
bioenergetic principles of health, and an ecological understanding
of man in relationship to the universe. It is also founded on a subtle holistic understanding of the interrelation between body and
mind, and between the person and the surrounding environment.
Harmony and balance are the keynotes of Chinese medicine. By
application of natural law, the Oriental Medical Doctor (OMD)
maintains the good health of his patients. Dr. Joseph Needham,
a respected authority on Chinese science and culture, translates
this passage from the *Nei Ching:*

> Huang Ti, the Yellow Emperor, once inquired of his court
> physician, Chi Po, 'I should like to know the Tao (way) of
> Acupuncture?' Chi Po replied, 'The first thing in this art and

mystery is that you must concentrate the mind on the patient
as a whole . . ."[3]

Historically, Chinese medicine is one of the most prominent
medical systems on this planet. It has strongly influenced traditional medicine in the Orient, especially Korea, Japan, and Vietnam. In contemporary China, the traditional medicine of herbs
and acupuncture is practiced in hospitals alongside conventional
Western medicine, and around the world this ancient tradition
is gaining new supporters. Although acupuncture is relatively new
to the United States, many European countries such as France and
Germany have been using acupuncture since the turn of the century. In France, acupuncture (and homeopathy) are taught in
several medical schools.

Today we are living in a medical renaissance. Western medicine has reached a pinnacle and is now becoming receptive to new
ideas. Holistic medicine is making a resurgence in modern industrial countries, and over the last decade acupuncture has received
much publicity. Newspapers, magazines, and television have focused their attention on this ancient healing art. Even modern
medical research journals are scrutinizing this medicine with increasing evidence that acupuncture does indeed work. Experts in
the field of acupuncture research include: Richard C. Chapman,
Ph.D., M.D., professor at the University of Washington, Department of Anesthesiology, and Bruce Pomeranz, M.D., Ph.D.,
neurosurgeon and professor at the University of Toronto. Dr.
Pomeranz emphatically states:

> I can't see a better solution to long term chronic pain. There
> is no question in my mind that [acupuncture] is safer than surgery
> or drugs because it stimulates the natural chemical changes of
> the body.[4]

Dr. Pomeranz's research and interest with acupuncture has
resulted in a book, *Acupuncture: Textbook and Atlas*. In the introduction, he surveys 228 pertinent articles relating to the efficacy
and explanation of acupuncture.

When one is first confronted with acupuncture, it seems rather unbelievable that tiny needles inserted just under the skin can actually promote healing. When it was first introduced into America, acupuncture was denounced on the grounds that it lacked scientific validation—a situation that is rapidly changing. In this century, great minds such as Aldous Huxley have pondered this curious phenomenon:

> Within our system of explanations there is no reason why the needleprick should be followed by an improvement of the liver function. Therefore we say that it cannot happen. The only trouble with this argument is that as a matter of empirical fact, it does happen. Inserted at precisely the right point, a needle in the foot affects the function of the liver.[5]

Years ago, when we first started our study of acupuncture, people wanted to know, "Does acupuncture work?" Nowadays we more frequently hear, "How does it work?" As of yet, no one really knows the answer to this question. At present there is a flood of theories from both the East and West, some with more justification than others. Scientists have conclusively demonstrated that the nervous system is involved, but the actual process remains a mystery.

The weight of Western research indicates that acupuncture works by stimulating the nerve trunks near the acupuncture points. For example, Dr. Pomeranz has shown that the stimulation of Large Intestine-4 (*Ho Ku*) on laboratory animals triggers the pituitary to release endorphin, a hormone 5,000 times stronger than heroin. If, however, the radial nerve is severed above this point, there is no release of this hormone.[6]

The "gate theory," a popular Western attempt to explain acupuncture, postulates that needle stimulation jams nerve impulses, preventing pain signals from reaching the brain. Although possibly true, the gate theory is rather limited and does not adequately explain how acupuncture promotes healing. The architects of this theory do not consider traditional Chinese medical knowledge worth their attention.

Current research more in tune with Chinese medical philosophy includes that of Robert Becker, M.D. Dr. Becker has succeeded in mapping out meridian flows and their acupuncture points, and has determined their specific rhythmic pulses which consist of a fifteen minute pulsation cycle overlapping a longer cycle of twenty-four hours. Becker has also discovered that these meridians conduct a current and hypothesizes that the perineural system acts as the conductor.[7]

Claude Darras, a French medical doctor, has conducted interesting experiments in an attempt to trace the physical effects of acupuncture. When a radioactive isotope is injected into an acupuncture point, it moves away from the point in a predictable path, following no known anatomical pathways but rather specific acupuncture meridians. Isotopes injected into nonacupuncture point sites do not reproduce this specific motion. Also, when the isotope ceases to move, its movement can be restimulated by needling the point directly beneath the injection.[8]

Dr. Bjorn Nordenstrom speculates that his discovery of biologically-closed electrical circuits may be the key to the puzzle of acupuncture.[9] And yet another theory recently postulated by the scientific community is the possibility of unknown pathways in the nervous system linking various parts of the body. If this does prove true, then it will become very clear how a tiny needle stimulating a point on the foot would influence the liver. The Chinese have always maintained that the pathways of *chi* do link parts of the body. Later, it will be worthwhile to discuss these concepts in greater detail.

Present-day scientific research, as we have previously explained, adheres to what we call "the mechanistic model." This model serves as the guideline for current scientific thought and practice. The microscope offers a wonderful analogy into the nature of this approach, revealing its strengths and weaknesses. The microscope is undeniably one of the great tools of modern science, without which the bulk of biology and medicine would not have evolved. But the microscope is also symbolic of the Western tendency towards over-specialization; we become so intent on the part that we miss the whole. Imagine using the microscope to determine that the animal before you is an elephant! As ridiculous as this seems, there are actually such parallels found in Western science.[10]

Because of this reflexive adherence to methodological dogma, there is an attempt to squeeze all acupuncture research into the standard biochemical model. This kind of biochemical research is, of course, necessary and productive, but until now it has dealt with acupuncture on a simplistic level, primarily as a painkiller. Even worse, many studies of acupuncture have been conducted by scientists who have no understanding of Chinese medical philosophy. Fortunately, this situation is changing, as scientists at last begin to glimpse the underlying wisdom of the East.

From quantum physics has emerged a new view of the universe, the "holographic paradigm." This innovative model was originally proposed by physicist David Bohm, whose text on quantum physics, *Quantum Theory*, is required reading for many aspiring physicists. A hologram is an intriguing phenomenon. A special photographic technique for creating three-dimensional pictures, it is unique in the sense that a broken segment contains all the information necessary to reproduce the total picture. Holographic theory proposes that much of the universe, including the brain, works on a similar principle. This holistic model suggests startling new concepts: for instance, "holoverse" for universe, and "holomotion" rather than time. It is apparent that holographic theory is related to the Eastern holistic perspectives of the universe.

Many scientists, understanding the limitations of the Newton model, are following this trend toward Western recognition of ancient Oriental wisdom. Neils Bohr, co-developer of the famous "Copenhagen interpretation of quantum physics," is widely considered one of the greatest minds since Isaac Newton. When Dr. Bohr was knighted for his outstanding scientific achievements in science, he chose for his coat of arms the Taoist monad—the *yin/yang* symbol—to emphasize his respect for Chinese philosophy. Of mechanistic thought, Bohr states:

> The great extension of our experience in recent years has brought to light the insufficiency of our simple mechanical concepts and, as a consequence, has shaken the foundation on which our customary interpretation of observation was based.[11]

Chinese medicine is based on a concept of the body as a unified energy system. This energy is the basis of all life. It is the organizational force behind all body processes and functions, including healing. *Chi* precedes and includes the nervous system. The clue to understanding how acupuncture works is found within the nature of *chi*, what it is and how it works.

Chinese medical theory claims that disease is caused by a blockage or weakness of *chi*, thus upsetting the normal homeostasis. If this energy imbalance is allowed to continue, a physical change in the tissue will occur, resulting in the pathological symptoms which are the focus of modern medical research and treatment.

WEAK CHI ————————→ TISSUE CHANGE = PATHOLOGY
(or blocked)   (yields)   (Western disease entity)

How does the Chinese physician discern this energy imbalance? While this question will be answered more fully in the next chapter, the OMD relies on keen observational skills and sensitive palpation techniques that have been handed down through generations of practitioners. Over the centuries the understanding has evolved that these irregularities in life energy manifest themselves in distinct patterns, which we refer to as "patterns of disharmony."

Because these patterns are derived from the literal translation of poetic intentions, they often have odd, even outlandish-sounding names. One of the models used for these descriptions is ecologically based, reflecting the Oriental concept of the body as an integrated, internal environment. DAMPNESS, HEAT, and WIND,[12] for example, are expressions which utilize this environmental paradigm to portray patterns of disharmony. Other patterns, more complex, refer to obtuse energy relationships (such as DEFICIENT KIDNEY JING) which require years of study to understand fully. Please do not dismiss these disharmony patterns as primitive or archaic without full investigation.

Since these diagnoses explain qualities of energy, it should be obvious that the terminology would be radically different from that of Western medicine. The OMD is trained to make precise statements regarding the individual's specific energetic imbalance.

This statement is the diagnosis and implies the treatment. For these reasons, Oriental medicine can recognize and treat long before there is pathological tissue damage, thus distinguishing it as a true preventative medicine.

Normal Western diagnostic terms such as "hypertension," "hepatitis," or "conjunctivitis" are not considered diagnoses, but rather *symptoms* of a deeper underlying disorder. For example, the above symptoms could be indicators of a disturbance in the *liver* energy, possibly LIVER YANG RISING or LIVER FIRE BLAZING. These diagnoses, while they do sound strange, are in fact graphic representations of disharmony patterns. They describe the totality of a person's condition, emphasizing the patient's overall energy and internal environment.

These energetic patterns are symbolic representations of a person's energy imbalance. This energy field is very real, like the force fields surrounding magnets or the earth. The Chinese have empirically dissected this field into distinct lines which radiate through and around the body. As these lines of (bio)force flow through their respective organs and limbs, they are known as "meridians of acupuncture." Acupuncture works by directly manipulating this living current and inducing a state of equilibrium. Acupuncture points along these meridians are the control stations where this energy is regulated. And as we have already pointed out, scientific evidence for these acupuncture points and meridians continues to mount.

What causes the *chi* to become weak or imbalanced? There are many possible origins; Chinese medicine divides them into "internal," "external," and "miscellaneous" causes. External causes derive from accidents and from environmental influences, like cold or damp, which the Chinese call "external evils." Internal causes are precipitated by many factors, including stress and diet. Dietary imbalances are a key consideration in Chinese medicine because different kinds of food can adversely affect the internal environment. For example, if a person consumes a predominance of cold foods (such as salads, ice cream, or chilled foods) this will result in an overcooling condition in the body which in turn can produce a variety of unpleasant symptoms; if one eats a predominance of processed, devitalized food products, the body will suffer from *chi* deficiency.

"Stress" is a broad term that encompasses many factors. Stress can come from traffic jams, over-anxious bosses, marital conflicts and any of the other pressures of life. People respond to stress by tensing their muscles. If this tension becomes pronounced, the flow of *chi* through the body becomes restricted. When this tension becomes severe, it can produce an "armoring" around the body which can actually block the flow of energy to different parts of the body. For this reason meditation, relaxation exercises, and exercise are important to reopen this flow of energy through the muscles. Taoists, the ancient monks who developed acupuncture, have developed specific meditations to open and control the various energy pathways in the body. Acupuncture is reknowned for its beneficial effect on stress and tension.

After the oriental medical diagnosis is determined, the treatment is directed at restoring the imbalance in the person's energy system, utilizing the eight branches either singularly or in combination. For example, a combination of herbs and acupuncture might be applied. The intent is to harmonize and balance the *chi* in the different systems and organs by application of specific methods, according to various "energetic laws": *yin* and *yang*, the eight principles, the five phases, and the six layers.

Chinese medicine is a medical science based on thousands of years of observations, clinical experimentation, and critical thinking. Specific stimuli applied by properly-trained professionals to specific sites on the body can and do regulate health. The remainder of this chapter and the next will be devoted to the philosophy, history, and application of Chinese medicine.

Chinese Thought and Language: A Holisitic Perspective

There is a great chasm between the East and the West. If the concepts from Eastern and Western culture are ever truly to merge, it can only happen by understanding the substantial differences in languages and thought processes between these two societies. Chinese medicine in the West suffers from this chasm because of the many inherent difficulties in translating even one book, much less the vast body of literature accumulated over thirty centuries.

Perhaps the best place to start is with a comparison between inductive and deductive logic. For simplicity, we begin with the assumption that inductive logic corresponds to Eastern thought and right-hemispheric brain processes, and that deductive logic corresponds to Western thought and left-hemispheric brain processes. Table 3 illustrates these correspondences, which we will now attempt to validate.

Deductive logic is linear in nature. It proceeds from premise to conclusion, from point A to point B, much in the same way that we construct a word from our alphabet, letter by letter. Letters of the alphabet can be seen as similar to premises, and words become their conclusions. Table 4 is a typical example of deductive logic.

Although scientists are currently postulating that the brain works in some sort of holographic manner, it is still useful and valid to discuss left- and right-brain processes, remembering that they are only statistical and most certainly not absolute. The Kahuna priests of Hawaii categorized these functions as "lower" and "higher" mind, which is perhaps a more accurate terminology. At any rate, it is convenient for us to visualize the right and left brain as categories for tabulating different types of brain function. For instance, it is known that in most brains the left hemisphere predominantly controls deductive functions—linear flow of information, mathematics, and so on. From Table 3 it is easy to see that these left brain processes dominate in Western culture, leading to an imbalance—we are too analytical. Inductive logic, on the other hand, corresponds to functions that predominate on the right hemisphere of the brain, involving creative and intuitive processes that are intrinsically holistic. Much art, like painting and poetry, is inductive in nature because it stems from an understanding of the whole. Patterns, relationships, and symbols can all be aspects of inductive creativity. A symbol is a concrete image that signifies

Table 3: Left and Right Brain Related Processes

LEFT BRAIN	RIGHT BRAIN
TIME	SPACE
LINEAR FLOWS	SPACIAL RELATIONSHIPS
OF INFORMATION	
Sequential processing (writing letter by letter to make a word; word by word to make a sentence; etc.)	Simultaneous processing (juggling; playing the piano; driving a race car; et. al.)
Analysis (bit by bit)	Gestalt (patterned wholes)
Verbal Memory	Non-verbal memory (music, tempo, movement)
Mathematics	Geometry
Technical	Creative
Digital	Analog
Analytic	Synthetic
Historic	Timeless
DEDUCTION	INDUCTION
Causal	Holistic
Rational	Intuitive
Deductive	Analogous
WESTERN THOUGHT	EASTERN THOUGHT
Linear	Circular
YANG	YIN

Table 4: Deductive Logic

Premise	All birds have feathers	(true)
Premise	All sparrows are birds	(true)
Conclusion	Therefore all sparrows have feathers	(true)

a whole concept or ideal (think of all the symbology conveyed by the American flag).

Inductive reasoning is based on past experiences and empirical observations. It must be emphasized that inductive arguments do not prove their conclusions; deductive arguments, however, do. Induction relies on statistical evidence or probable outcomes. You are using inductive reasoning when you buy tomatoes from a store. From past experience, you know the best tomatoes are a particular color, texture, and firmness. However, choosing a tomato that meets these requirements doesn't necessarily insure a good-tasting tomato. There is always the possibility that after exercising these precautions, it will be rotten inside. But it is certain that by following these guidelines, one will buy a greater percentage of superior tasting tomatoes. With induction, like statistics, the larger the sample the stronger the argument. For this reason, we view inductive sciences as being somewhat statistical.

Chinese medicine and homeopathy are examples of what we call inductive sciences (sciences that rely more predominantly on inductive logic). Their very foundations are rooted in empirical observations and cyclical processes, each relying to some degree on holistic appraisal (a right-brain function). These sciences are not like our familiar Western sciences which are entrenched in the hard, cold facts of deductive logic. This does not mean, however, that inductive sciences are in some way inferior; they are not. Both inductive and deductive methodologies have their value. In the final estimate, it is impossible to separate induction and deduction (like *yin* and *yang*) because one cannot exist without the other, and even deductive facts are inspired at some point by inductive reasoning. Vicki Cobb, a logician, says, "Inductive reasoning is at the very core of the discovery of scientific truth." [13]

We are all familiar with the stories of the great scientists who, in a flash of inspiration, began work on some marvelous new discovery. Everyone has heard the proverbial story of Newton's flash of intuition when an apple fell on him while he was pondering the universe. From that moment, it is said, he conceived his monumental inspiration, the universal law of gravity. James Watson, co-discoverer of the DNA helix, the code of genetics, came upon its unique spiral form while daydreaming during a Marlene Dietrich movie. These occurrences are part of the right brain's amazing capacity for synthesis and generation of images. These two events are analogous to what happens when a person experiences a near-death situation and sees his entire life flash before his eyes. This is a right-brain capacity to see the whole—the totality—at one instant (while the left brain processes sequential information one bit at a time).

The Chinese language is based on a system of imagery, while Western languages are based on a system of linear bits. Now we are on the verge of a new frontier where both of these vital perspectives can be understood. In her book, *The Possible Human*, psychologist Jean Houston presents exercises designed to integrate and coordinate functions of the right and left brain. Elsewhere, researcher and author Robert Monroe of The Monroe Institute has developed an evolutionary sound technique known as "Hemisync," which empirically balances the left and right brain. The term "whole brain" is becoming a key phrase in contemporary literature.

As we noted in the previous chapter, the circle (O) and the straight line (——) are wonderful symbols illustrating the inherent differences between Eastern and Western thought, respectively. Western research substantiates this analogy; scientists have discovered that left-brain neurons statistically control functions relating to time (a more linear process), while right-brain neurons statistically control functions that relate to spatial perception—space (a more circular, holistic process).[14]

A circle, therefore, becomes a crucial key to understanding inductive logic, Chinese thought, and right-brain activities. The circle represents the "whole"—a complete statement, the totality. It is for this reason that induction is so difficult to explain (deduction only required half a page), and why the essence of Chinese philosophy is so elusive. Peter Eckman, a medical doctor who practices acupuncture, discusses this dilemma:

. . . everything in Oriental medicine is part of a circular process; that's why the Tao is symbolized by a circle.
As we're trying to break off a chunk of it [Chinese medicine is represented by the circle] and analyze it and teach
it from one or another perspective, inevitably what's going to happen, in the middle of it, I will get stuck and
need to talk about something else because that's part of
what explains this edge of the circle (here). So I need to
talk about what's over there and likewise, if I tried to
break in over there I'd have to talk about what's over
here . . . [15]

With all this discussion of inductive/deductive reasoning,
right/left-brain thinking, and circular/linear processes, one might
wonder: Within the larger context of this "merging" process, where
is all of this leading us? What greater whole or truth is being realized? We don't profess to know, but perhaps herein lie the secrets
to space/time itself.

Leaving these philosophical questions behind, let's now discuss
the Chinese language and its translation quagmire. Chinese, in
diametric contrast to Western languages, is a pictorial, symbolic
language. These poetic, evocative, linguistic qualities are directly
responsible for its variant emphasis, making Chinese thought more
inductive than Western. Each Chinese word is actually a character,
and each character—directly derived from a picture (pictogram)
or image (ideogram)—is capable of conveying vast meanings and
nuances of thought which are impossible in our language. Even a
simple sentence in Chinese can resound with allusion and imagery.
For instance, a sentence from an old Chinese text is translated,
"The *chi* should be *excited*, the spirit internally gathered." Of the
word *excited*, this translator carefully notes, "The Chinese character representing the word *excited* actually has the connotation:
if all the oceans of the world were gathered into a box and the
box was jiggled, the water would slosh back and forth."[16] From
this example one glimpses the vast quantities of information that
can be stored in one simple ideogram.

Furthermore, individual pictorial images can be combined
to convey more complex ideas. From this crude prehistoric pic-

ture of a tree (𝖸) was refined the Chinese character for tree (木), a pictogram. The combination of two trees (林) expresses the idea of forest, an ideogram. Another pictogram (日), the sun was refined from this prehistoric picture (⊙). The combination of these two pictograms, "the sun" and "the tree," produces the ideogram for "the east" (東)—the sun seen peeking through the trees.

As we have mentioned, the potential for storing extensive information within a single character is only one of the many problems faced by the translator of Chinese (and his readers). There are also major difficulties in the treatment of Chinese intonation, transliteration, and semantics. Let's look at each of these problems now.

The task of translating intonation, while similar to the one just discussed, is alien to Western languages; most translators regrettably neglect to account for this essential linguistic element. It is the omission of intonation that creates such a nightmare of frustration and confusion for the casual reader of translated Chinese literature. If you have ever heard the Chinese language spoken you cannot help but notice its beautiful sing-song quality. In fact, its words *are* sung; depending on the type of rising or falling note expressed, the same phonetic sound can represent several completely separate words. In Chinese, such distinctions present no problems, for each separate intonation (of a phonetic sound) has its own unique character, a picture which conveys its own multiplicity of meanings (while we are usually left with a highly inaccurate phonetic equivalent). For instance, our familiar expression for the positive duality, *yang*, sung another way means sheep. How, without proper intonation marks, could one ever be sure of the correct meaning?

The process of translating Chinese characters into phonetic equivalents is called "transliteration." Unfortunately, there are many systems of transliteration which greatly complicates this linguistic puzzle. Since each style of transliteration has its own method of spelling, this results in many different spellings for the same phonetic sound. For instance, the word *chi* is also spelled "*qi*" and "*ji*." The capital of China, "Peking," is also spelled "Beijing" and "Beiqing." All of this depends on which system you are using (and we're not even including the intonation marks). Furthermore, it should be kept in mind that all of these systems are in essence artificial. Anyone familiar with the computer world can easily sympathize, for the task of transliteration poses as many inherent problems as a computer engineer faces when attempting to translate an analog signal to a digital code. (An analog signal is created by varying the voltage of an otherwise constant current, while digital varies the current of an otherwise constant voltage by turning it on and off in Morse Code fashion.) Sounds difficult? It is! Now imagine attempting to compare notes from several translated Chinese sources.

The next area of concern, semantics, is of course a problem for any historical translator. Semantics is the study of meaning in language, particularly with regard to its historical change. It is virtually impossible to understand the original intention of an author if the connotations and denotations of a word in relationship to the era are not implicitly understood. This is particularly difficult for the translator of ancient Chinese, not only as a result of all the previously discussed cultural differences, but also because of the extreme length of time involved, Chinese being the oldest intact language.

In fact for true accuracy the ideal translator or writer of Chinese medicine would need a thorough understanding of all the above; English and all its intricacies; as well as the subject itself—Chinese medicine. This is, exactly, what makes authors such as Kaptchuk, Bensky, and Gamble so successful.

History

Like her boundaries, China's history is one of constant change, ebbing and flowing, a mighty tidal river against the backdrop of time. Even in her infancy, several thousand years before Christ, primitive tribes on the northern plains were continually quarreling and feuding. Over the centuries, the Chin tribe eventually gained the advantage and conquered the other major tribes, creating the first unification in 221 B.C. Corrupt from the beginning, the Chin dynasty lasted a mere fourteen years.

Supported by the people, the Han tribe swiftly took over, setting the stage for the rhythmic pulsations of Chinese history. Throughout Chinese history, one sees this basic cycle of unification, struggle, disintegration, then unification. Distinct periods of government in Chinese history are marked by a system of dynasties. For instance, the present dynasty—the People's Republic—is but a brief speck of dust in China's 5000-year history, and in time it too will disappear.

In the West, we often perceive the Chinese as an ignorant race of barbarians because our knowledge of their history and culture is somewhat shallow. But examination reveals that their history has been highlighted by many brilliant epochs of civilization. Their inventions include the compass, in 3 B.C.; the suspension bridge, in 600 A.D.; and gun powder, in 1100 A.D.; all prior to their discovery in the west.[17] Before the birth of Christ, the Chinese had accomplished marvelous feats of engineering. The China Wall, one of the great wonders of the world, is over 1600 miles long and was built over very rugged terrain. Much of China's complex irrigation system, built as far back as the third century B.C., is still in use.[18] Its construction required advanced knowledge of hydraulics.

The Chinese invented paper, and were printing books long before the West. These ancient manuscripts, on display in museums around the world, are masterpieces of skill and organization. China, the first producer of silk, still counts it as one of its major exports along with teas and spices.

Chinese religion, art, and philosophy are world reknowned for their refinement and achievement. Chinese culture was for centuries the mother of younger countries such as Korea and Japan. Chinese medicine, acupuncture, and herbs traveled to these countries where they are still in use. Chinese ceramics and paintings are well loved around the world for their delicate beauty and fine craftsmanship. Today, in America, there is increasing interest in ancient Chinese ideas, with the proliferation of books on Taoism, the numerous martial arts schools, and, of course, acupuncture.

The history of Chinese medicine is as ancient as the country itself. Early legends abound with tales of great men like Shen Nung (3494 B.C.), the first practitioner known to have used herbs therapeutically, and Huang Ti, the Yellow Emperor (2674 B.C.), often considered the founder of Chinese medicine. The annals of this medicine are filled with countless healers whose lives were a tribute to their profession. It is somewhat remarkable to observe the medical discoveries and advancements that occurred in China long before their appearance in the West. For instance, the Chinese were aware of the circulation of blood hundreds of years before its discovery by William Harvey in 1628.[19]

Sun Si Mao (581–682 A.D.), a truly great medical scholar by any standards, recognized pulmonary tuberculosis as a lung disorder. He understood that it was an infectious disease of the lung viscera, a new concept in his time.[20] Another of Sun Si Mao's outstanding contributions to medicine was the realization that goiter was a disease of malnutrition. For this illness he prescribed the thyroid glands from a sheep or a deer—both rich in iodine. Among his many other advances, he promoted proper hygiene, pediatric care, and diet therapy.[21]

Huo To, one of the first recorded surgeons in history, performed surgery as early as the second century, A.D.[22] Another pioneer physician, Zhang Zhong-jing (142–220 A.D.), witnessed the death of many relatives during a severe epidemic, a tragedy that inspired him to study medicine. Zhang's book on treating febrile and epidemic diseases is a landmark in Chinese history.[23]

The dedication, perseverance, and skill of these healers is often inspiring. One such doctor was Chu Tan Chi (1281–1358 A.D.). Chu was known far and wide for his humanitarian nature, often treating poor patients for no charge. He would visit patients in distant places, carrying drugs and treating them on their farms.[24]

Li Shi-zhen, the great herbalist, devoted his entire life to producing his massive materia medica of natural drugs which was not published until three years after his death in 1593. This book, still used, consists of sixteen volumes and includes 1,893 medicinal substances from botanical, zoological and mineral sources.[25]

As it is practiced today, Chinese medicine is the result of centuries of accumulated effort by generations of great physicians. Like any other serious medical system, Chinese medicine takes years to master. Traditionally, it was taught in long arduous apprenticeship. This notion that anyone—including medical doctors—can learn this medicine in a brief intensive course is totally absurd. Would you trust a person who had only taken a two-week course in surgery to operate on you? Chinese medicine requires mastery of its medical facts and philosophy; most importantly, it entails extensive clinical experience. Repeated practical experience is the only way to understand this healing science. It is also necessary for any sincere student to intern with an accomplished Eastern doctor if he wishes to master this profession.

In conclusion to this chapter, we should mention the impact Western medicine has made on China.[26] During the beginning of this century, with the influx of Western medicine and the Westernization of China, the traditional art was ignored. The eager, modern Chinese considered it part of an antiquated past. However, Chairman Mao, in one of his more inspired actions, revived and restored the traditional medicine during the 1950's. During Mao's incredible survival on the "long march" in his battle with Chiang Kai-shek, his army was cut off from its Western medical supplies for several years. Out of necessity, the troops resorted to their traditional medicine which still flourished in spite of legal sanctions against its practice. Mao and his generals were impressed with the results. It was this direct experience that spurred the enthusiastic support of traditional herbalists and acupuncturists when he came to power. Mao created a new type of national hero when his vision of an army of health practitioners was realized in the historic "barefoot doctor" campaign. Today in China, Eastern and Western medicine are often practiced side by side; at the entrance to some Chinese hospitals the patient can turn left or right, depending on which kind of treatment he desires: Western or Eastern. But as in the West, many "modern" Chinese doctors, trained solely in biochemical medicine, raise their noses at the traditional arts of herbalism and acupuncture, a sad trait considering the richness of their medical heritage. Overall, however, the Chinese, whether medically trained or not, have a great respect for their traditional medicine because they know it works.

5

Ancient Medicine for a Modern World

"Of all things in the universe, human beings are most precious."

Confucius

Chinese medicine, like other inductive sciences, seems initially impossible to learn. This confusion lies within the circular nature of this type of system: Where does a circle start and exactly how do you convey the totality of this complex concept with all its intricate relationships? Western sciences, intrinsically more deductive, are far simpler to explain. Facts are stacked upon facts in a linear fashion to get from point A to point B. On the other hand, because inductive systems are holistic in nature, one must grasp the totality of the picture before it can be of real value; this effort requires patience and observation. With these obstacles in mind, we will attempt to explain Chinese medicine as clearly as possible.

In the West we are too often consumed by the desire to know "why." Western thinking from Aristotle's time has been dominated by this idea of causation. Chinese thought, however, is more concerned with observing the synchronicity of nature. "The key word in Chinese thought is order and above all *pattern*."[1] To the Chinese, nature reveals herself to the person who takes time to watch her unfold in the inevitable cycles of movement and change.

The Oriental medical doctor (OMD) learns to observe his patients through the changing patterns of health and disease. He must implicitly understand the relationship of man to the cosmos, how this affects man's *chi,* and how this *chi* flows through the body. He must be able to recognize the signs that indicate imbalances and distortions in this energy flow. Most importantly, he must discern from these signs and symptoms the particular pattern of disharmony. This is the goal of diagnosis and the key to cure. This goal, as you can well imagine, is no easy matter. The first step is a thorough and fundamental understanding of *yin* and *yang.*

Yin and *Yang*

Yin and *yang* are descriptive terms for classifying universal polar relationships. *Yin* is relatively more negative, *yang* more positive. (Notice the use of the word "relatively" here; just as with right- and left-brain concepts, *yin* and *yang* are not absolutes.) Everything in the universe is in some type of polar relationship. In the human body there are countless examples of the *yin/yang* relationship, such as the electrolytic balance between sodium and potassium ions, or the rhythmic pulsation of the heart and respiration. Just as magnets, batteries, and other electrical devices have their obvious polarities, so do intangible concepts: "beauty" implies its opposite, "ugly"; dirty implies clean; and so on. Likewise, all processes and manifestations in the universe are in dynamic flux between *yin* and *yang.* In Table 5, we list a few common examples.

The subtle symbology of *yin* and *yang* is most ingeniously expressed in the Taoist monad, sometimes referred to as a *syzygy.*

     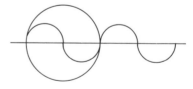

The outer circle represents the *tao* ("the one," "the path," or "the totality"). This circle is divided in half by a sine wave whose focal points are represented by two contrasting black and white dots.

The top half is black, symbolizing *yin;* the bottom, white,

Table 5

YIN	YANG
moon	sun
night	day
cold	hot
water	fire
dark	light
woman	man
interior	exterior
chronic	acute
moist	dry
structure	action
nourishment	growth
contractive	expansive
centripetal	centrifugal
passive	aggressive
south pole	north pole
neutron	electron
blood	*chi*
(−)	(+)

symbolizing *yang*. Notice how gracefully they flow into each other: the *yang* rising into the *yin*, the *yin* sinking into the *yang*, illustrating their paradoxical unity yet separateness. *Yin* cannot exist without *yang*, and vice-versa; they are mutually dependent, and one is not better or worse than the other. *Yin* and *yang* are in a constant state of flux and transformation, as repeated by the two contrasting dots (focal points). These dots symbolize a subtle aspect of Taoist philosophy which states, "Nothing in the universe is entirely *yin* or *yang*. One cannot exist without the other. Within *yin* there is always the seed of *yang* and within *yang* there is always the seed of *yin*."[2]

As anything in the universe approaches absolute *yin* or *yang*, it is transformed into its opposite. The more extreme the situation, the faster and more drastic this transformation. Absolute *yin* or *yang* is impossible.

In the clinic we see verifications of these principles. An extremely *yang* patient, suffering from high blood pressure and headaches, suddenly has a stroke and becomes paralyzed—extreme *yang* is transformed into *yin*. Chronically ill patients will often exhibit a curious phenomenon: Just before death, they will improve dramatically and an appearance of vitality will return, like a candle flickering brightly before it goes out. This is *yin* momentarily transforming to *yang*.

Yin and *yang* are usually considered a dualistic concept; however, an in-depth study reveals that there are trinary overtones to Taoist philosophy. The *yin/yang* symbol itself reveals this implied third element. When *yin* and *yang* come together in this symbol they are used to represent the totality of the universe— the *Tao*. Oscar Brunler, M.D., illustrates this feature succinctly:

> Let us for a fleeting moment look at some of the basic laws which we use in all spheres of science. These laws are the foundation stones and without them we cannot build up anything of value.
>
> The law of polarity may be called the first and the fundamental law of all creation. Only man and woman together can create a child. Only a positive and a negative electric current can produce an electric light. Only an acid (positive) and an alkali (negative) can produce a chemical compound. Only the joining of the two—the positive and the negative—can create a new manifestation.
>
> All attempts to discard this basic law and to hope for results without using it is a waste of time and energy. Two acids cannot combine and form a new chemical compoung. Two positive currents cannot produce a light. Two positive poles of a magnet repel each other. The whole of creation is the joining of two forces of an opposite and complementary nature or an opposite polarity. When these two forces join creation takes place. In every sphere of science we see that this basic law manifests itself.[3]

Brunler was not the first to realize these trialistic concepts concerning universal law. In the East, Taoist sages understood these concepts centuries ago, and in the West, Descartes reasoned the existence of God as a third element from the dualistic concepts of mind and matter (a polarity).[4] It is interesting that Oriental philosophers discerned this fact inductively while Western philosophers used a deductive approach to reach the same conclusion.

Because we know that all forms of energy oscillate between negative and positive polarities (*yin* and *yang*), and we also know (from Albert Einstein) that matter too is energy, this oscillation principle now becomes a fundamental fact of the universe. Everything in the universe is but a vibration. No wonder many modern physicists are excited about Taoist philosophy!

Diagnosis

A correct diagnosis is crucial to the success of any treatment, no matter what the modality. Conventional medicine diagnoses the visible pathology. It is usually this specific pathology that is considered the cause of the illness. Bioenergetic medicine, in contrast, determines a pattern of disharmony from the totality of symptoms. It is this disharmony that is considered the source of the disease.

Oriental medical doctors consider most Western disease categories (migraines, asthma, ulcer, etc.) to be symptoms of a larger pattern of disorder. In order to treat the whole person, the totality of symptoms must be examined to determine the picture of the disharmony. This determination is essential to initiate the healing process.

The Oriental medical doctor begins his diagnosis from the moment he greets his patient. Like a detective, he must recognize the subtle clues and hints in the tone of voice, gait, posture, facial expression, complexion, and peculiar mannerisms. All of these data (and more) provide invaluable clues on which to base the diagnosis. This type of doctor closely scrutinizes his patient with his own senses: sight, hearing, touch, and even smell. He also takes a complete medical history. All this information is integrated and forms what is called a "pattern of disharmony." These patterns, which we are going to discuss in detail, are ascertained using the following

energetic parameters: *yin* and *yang;* the twelve meridians; the eight
therapeutic principles; the five phases; and the six energetic layers.
These parameters are evaluated according to an ancient Chinese
medical traditional known as "the four examinations."

The Four Examinations

Chinese diagnostic procedure is firmly rooted in an ancient tradition: "the four examinations." The four examinations
were formally introduced in the fourth century B.C. by Pien Chueh,
the first Chinese physician of historical significance. Because of
his great reputation as a healer, Pien Cheuh's method of evaluating
his patients was recorded and passed along for posterity.[5] So simple and yet so ingenious is this procedure that it is still standard
operating procedure for the Chinese physician. Few changes have
been made in the basic method in its 2000-year history. This is
a technique designed to observe the whole patient, utilizing the
physician's senses. The four examinations are: 1) looking; 2) listening (and smelling); 3) asking; and 4) touching. While examining
the patient, the doctor is simultaneously classifying everything in
terms of *yin* and *yang,* eight principles, five phases, and the six
layers.

Looking

"Looking" is the visual inspection of the patient, and
it starts from the moment the patient enters the office. The list
of specific observations is rather long. Naturally, one looks at the
face, the expression, the posture, and all the minutiae of detail that
make the person unique. Probably the single most important visual
examination is looking at the tongue. As unlikely as it might seem,
the tongue can reveal a wealth of information regarding the patient's health. The tongue, the visible portion of the digestive tract,
reflects the basic "climate" of the internal environment: Is the internal climate hot, cold, damp, deficient, excessive, or imbalanced
in some other way? In our clinic, we are constantly amazed at
the individual variations of the tongue, and our patients are equally

curious at our concern for their tongues. A "normal" tongue is light red and somewhat moist. A pale tongue can indicate a lack of bioenergy; a red tongue most likely signifies excess heat, whereas a puffy tongue points to an excess of fluids. Three basic tongue aspects are evaluated: the shape, the tongue body, and the coat.

Listening and Smelling

"Listening" and "smelling" are represented by the same character in Chinese and therefore are discussed together. The doctor listens carefully to the sound of the patient's voice as this is a reflection of his overall condition. A patient with a loud, brassy voice could have an excess condition, whereas a patient with a soft voice may be deficient. Smelling might seem somewhat ludicrous to the Westerner, but this is an example of the subtlety of Chinese medicine. Just as each person has a distinctive tongue or fingerprint, each person has his own characteristic odor which in sickness becomes more pronounced, depending on the nature of the illness. For example, a Chinese doctor can detect by smell if someone has a tendency to kidney problems.

Asking

"Asking" simply means taking the medical history. Generally, this process is more detailed than its Western counterpart, because the practitioner wants to discover the totality of the patient's condition. Besides the standard questions, the doctor might inquire about such odd details as the patient's seasonal preferences, his favorite food, and times of the day that he feels worst. How does this particular person respond to the external world—this is a key question in the doctor's mind.

Touching

"Touching," the last of the four exams, refers to the information the doctor receives through his fingers. Palpation for tender areas on the abdomen or along acupuncture meridians is one reliable diagnostic tool. However, the most important aspect of touching is the art of taking the pulse. This is perhaps the OMD's most valuable diagnostic tool, one that requires years of experience to master. Chinese pulse-taking involves a system of comparisons along the radial artery near the wrist. The pulse can be taken in other locations on the body, but the wrist is the most convenient and common. "Reading" the pulse brings the practitioner into contact with the "internal environment" of his patient because the quality of the blood flow reflects the internal condition. Besides "reading" subtle changes or distortions in the *chi* and *blood*, the doctor can also detect specific information about each organ/meridian system. Often, the good Chinese doctor can tell the patient where his weaknesses are before the patient describes them. This fact might seem implausible to the reader, but pulse-taking is a valuable diagnostic tool that can be validated by experience and training. While good pulse-taking is a wonderful diagnostic method, it is not infallible. The doctor must compile and integrate all his information before determining a final diagnosis.

Observing the tongue and taking the pulse are the two most important elements of the four examinations. In the Orient many books have been devoted over the centuries to these two subjects alone. At one time Western doctors relied more on the evidence of their own senses. We are all familiar with the image of the old-fashioned country physician who spent much time with his patients and studied them carefully. In current Western medicine, the tongue is virtually ignored and the pulse is only measured for its rate.

In Chinese medicine, however, there are twenty-eight basic pulse qualities to detect: "slow," "fast," "empty," "slippery," "wiry," and "irregular," to name a few. Each of these pulse qualities signifies a different disharmony, as does each of the various pictures of the tongue. The tongue and pulse are extremely sensitive barometers of the internal energy systems of the body. Chinese medicine has developed these examinations into a highly-refined art and science for determining functional disorders and subtle energetic disharmonies.

The Language of
Disharmony Patterns

"The language of Chinese Medicine, by definition, enables
the acupuncturist to decode symptoms and adopt a treatment under any circumstances, even if the patient presents
an illness with an unknown Western etiology, such as
multiple sclerosis; or a disease that is not recognized as
a pathological entity, as was the case with Barlow's disease
only twenty years ago; or other unnamed diseases."
                                        Yves Requena, M.D.[6]

Patterns of disharmony (also known as "Chinese energetics") are the Eastern equivalent to Western pathological diagnoses. Poetic as well as practical, these patterns are rooted in the
terms of its basic language (the acupuncture meridians, the eight
therapeutic principals, the five phases, the six energetical layers,
chi, and *blood* syndromes, and a few miscellaneous categories)
which constitute the vocabulary of Chinese energetical diagnosis.
In this section, we will discuss these major constituents, beginning
with the twelve meridians and concluding with examples describing the synthesis of these various terms to arrive at the diagnosis—
the pattern of disharmony.

The Meridians and
Organ Systems of Chinese Medicine

Chi, governed by *yin* and *yang*, flows like a current
through our bodies. It is essential that the physician understand
this flow so that he can harmonize the energy and thus restore
health. How does this living energy flow through our bodies? The
Chinese character *mo* (/ 脈) is commonly translated as "meridians." The meridians of acupuncture are the channels, or pathways
through which the *chi* flows in the body. These channels, illus-
trated on the acupuncture charts and now being recognized by
modern science, are reminiscent of a road map. In actuality, they
are three dimensional, and should be viewed as fields of force with

these hypothetical highways as their central foci. These fields are very similar to the lines of force surrounding the earth or a magnet. "Acupuncture points" are specific sites along these fields where the energy can be manipulated (similar to the fine-tuning knob on a television). There are many different kinds of acupuncture points. Some have regulating actions that are easy to understand: cooling, dispersing, warming, and tonifying. Others have complex energetic functions beyond the scope of this book. Herbs also have their own energetic function, many of which parallel or match those of acupuncture points. Both herbs and acupuncture are capable of regulating this flow of *chi*.

There are twelve primary meridians of acupuncture. Each serves as an energy conduit for a particular organ from which that meridian derives its name. For instance, the *chi* which flows through the *heart meridian* regulates that organ. There are six *yin* organ/meridian systems which are coupled to six *yang* systems, a crucial polar relationship. In addition to these twelve primary meridians, there are eight extraordinary meridians that are of clinical significance but will not be discussed in this book.

Table 6

	YIN ORGAN/ MERIDIAN SYSTEMS	YANG ORGAN/ MERIDIAN SYSTEMS
	(−)	(+)
1	Lungs	Large Intestine
2	Spleen	Stomach
3	Heart	Small Intestine
4	Kidney	Bladder
5	Pericardium	Triple Warmer
6	Liver	Gall Bladder

In Chinese medicine, we do *not* speak of individual organs like we find in Western medicine. This essential fact is so important that we will reiterate it several times in this book. Chinese medicine is based on an *energetic perspective* of the body/mind. The liver, for instance, is more than the isolated organ; it is also a meridian, and most critically a specific center of energy—in fact, it regulates the flow of *chi*. In Table 7 we see the basis of the Chinese organ/ meridian system. The noted Chinese scholar, Manfred Porkert, calls these systems "orbs," which he says are not organs but spheres of influence.[7] They not only include an organ and meridian but other psychic and emotional correspondences as well. For instance, the *liver meridian*, which controls the smooth flow of *chi* in the body, is also associated with irritability and anger. When we refer to the Chinese organ/meridian system, we will italicize it in order to distinguish it from the anatomical organ. In health, these "orbs" are in a state of balance; in disease, a state of imbalance is reflected in the various systems which the doctor reads and diagnoses. The Chinese "energetical" classification of the life energy and body is a unique holistic perspective of man from which we in the West have much to learn.

Table 7: The Chinese Organ/Meridian System: (Arranged in classical order of energy flow through the meridians of acupuncture)

ORGAN/ MERIDIANS	MAJOR FUNCTIONS	PRIMARY SYMPTOMOTOLOGY
Lungs	Rule the *chi* of the whole body; regulates respiration and skin.	Coughing, wheezing, asthma, dyspnea, bronchitis, sadness, fatigue.
Large Intestine	Rules waste removal.	Distended abdomen, constipation, dry stools, diarrhea.

Stomach	Rules the receiving and ripening of ingested foods and fluids.	Mouth sores, pain in epigastrium, belching, nausea, vomiting.
Spleen	Rules the transformation and transportation of food into *chi;* governs the blood.	Diarrhea, poor appetite, anemia, chronic hepatitis, hemophilia, lethargy, obsessions.
Heart	Rules the head and the blood vessels (houses the spirit).	Palpitations, insomnia, angina, depression.
Small Intestines	Separates the pure from the impure (turbid).	Vomiting, gas that won't pass, bloating, abdominal pain.
Bladder	Receives and excretes the urine.	Burning urine, sand in urine, incontinence.
Kidney	Stores the *jing* (reproductive energy); rules the bones; is the root of *yin* and *yang.*	Backache, chronic ear problems, chronic asthma, fears.
Pericardium	Protects and assists the heart.	Stress (especially with tightness in the chest), breast problems, anxiety.
Triple Warmer	The fire that controls the water (metabolism); regulates the three burning spaces (thoracic, digestive, urogenital).	Edema, stiff neck, tinnitus, irregularities in the three warmers.
Gall Bladder	Stores and secretes bile; assists the liver.	Bitter taste in mouth, nausea, jaundice, indecision.
Liver	Rules the free flowing and spreading of *chi;* stores the *blood.*	Anger, high blood pressure, headache, dizziness, red face, muscle spasm, retinitus, eye problems, pain in ribs.

The Eight Therapeutic Principles

The "eight principles" are a further refinement of *yin* and *yang*. This is a system of classifying symptoms into four polar compartments, comprising eight parameters: *yin* or *yang;* interior or exterior; cold or hot; and empty or full. Deceivingly simple, these eight parameters are of inestimable clinical value because they provide the first basic shape to the patient's pattern of disharmony. An exterior, hot, full condition is extremely *yang;* an interior, cold, empty condition is very *yin*. Between these two extremes exist the myriad conditions possible for man.

The terms "interior" and "exterior" refer to the origin and location of the illness. Chronic ailments are primarily interior in nature. Less critical ailments, like sprains and colds, are more exterior.

"Cold" and "hot" refer superficially to body temperature: Is the patient's temperature above normal or below? Such gross measurement, however, is not the only criterion required to make a diagnosis in this category, because there are many symptoms indicating a relative state of heat in the body that do not rely on measurement of body temperature. In Chinese medicine, fluctuations in the internal environment between hot and cold are far more subtly diagnosed than in Western medicine. A Chinese doctor often describes a patient as "overheating" when there are no signs of an elevated temperature. High blood pressure, acid indigestion, or vertigo can suggest overheating.

Of these four categories the last, "empty" and "full," is the most difficult to explain. Imagine a chronically ill person who has no energy for anything but to lie in bed all the time. This person is devoid of *chi* ("empty"). Conversely, visualize an energetic young athlete who comes down with a high fever and headache—this is a "full" or excess condition. In Table 8, we give a few examples of symptoms found in these various conditions. (Remember that in Chinese medicine, Western "diseases" are considered symptoms).

The eight principles are a guide for detecting basic imbalances that occur when the homeostasis is disrupted. Clinically the eight

Table 8

1)	YIN		YANG	
2) Interior:		Exterior:		
	ulcer		flu or cold	
	migraine		heat stroke	
	cancer		dysentery	
3) Cold:		Hot:		
	pale tongue		red tongue	
	slow movements		rapid jerky movements	
	clear urine		dark urine	
4) Empty:	(deficient)	Full:	(excess)	
	tired		robust	
	shallow breathing		coarse breathing	
	ashen face		red face	

principles are valuable and relatively easy to apply, but they are only the first step in creating a total picture of disharmony.

The Five Phases

The system of "the five phases," sometimes referred to as "the five elements," is a further elaboration of *yin* and *yang* and the eight principles. When the ancient Chinese philosopher/doctors observed the natural world, they noticed that the *yin* and *yang* movements evolve into five basic qualities of energy, which they named *wood, fire, earth, metal* and *water*. These words should not be taken too literally, since they are symbols of a deeper underlying quality of energy/movement.

Wood
"The seed begins to sprout"

Wood represents birth, the initial moving and growth phase. *Wood* is the season of spring, the energy of wind, and it is reflected in all growing matter. In the body we see the wood phase in the *liver* and *gall bladder*.

Fire
"The plant begins its rapid growth"

Fire represents the warming, rising qualities in nature, the surging upward phase (like childhood). *Fire* is the season of summer, the energy of heat (expansion), and results in air and gases. The *heart, small intestine*, (and other functions) relate to *fire*.

Earth
"The plant ripens and is harvested"

Earth represents mature fruition, the adult phase (the peak). It is the center; it is nourishing. The *earth* season is late summer when the plants are heavy with fruit; its energy is humid, and it results in the soil. The *spleen, pancreas*, and *stomach* relate to the *Earth phase*.

Metal
"The plant drops its seed and withers"

Metal represents the descending qualities of nature, the decline, the decaying. *Metal* is the season of fall, its energy is dry, and it is found in all inorganic matter. The *lungs* and *large intestine* are the *metal* functions in the body.

Water
"The seed rests in the ground waiting for spring and the rebirth"

Water represents the ending of a cycle, the death (and rebirth) phase. *Water* is the season of winter, the energy of cold (contraction), and manifests in all that is liquid. The *kidney* and *bladder* are the *water* organs in the body.

Table 9: Five-Phase Relationships

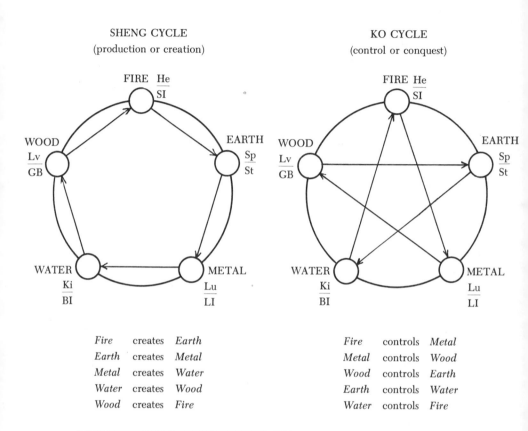

SHENG CYCLE
(production or creation)

KO CYCLE
(control or conquest)

Fire	creates	Earth
Earth	creates	*Metal*
Metal	creates	*Water*
Water	creates	*Wood*
Wood	creates	*Fire*

Fire	controls	*Metal*
Metal	controls	*Wood*
Wood	controls	*Earth*
Earth	controls	*Water*
Water	controls	*Fire*

The five phases find their correspondence in the body, mind, and diet. Looking at Tables 9 and 10, one sees how an imbalance of *water* (for example, *kidney* deficiency) can result in fears and phobias; how prolonged grief damages the *lungs* (which are *metal*) and hence the overall *chi;* or how eating too much sweet food injures the *spleen* (*earth*).

In a typical clinical situation, we might see a patient who is irritable and nervous, subject to headaches and occasional de-

Table 10: Five-Phase Correspondence

PHASE	WOOD	FIRE	EARTH	METAL	WATER
Season	Spring	Summer	Midsummer	Autumn	Winter
Direction	East	South	Center	West	North
Weather	Wind	Heat	Dampness	Dryness	Cold
Color	Green	Red	Yellow	White	Blue
Yin Organ	Liver	Heart	Spleen	Lungs	Kidneys
Yang Organ	Gallbladder	Small Intestine	Stomach	Large Intestine	Bladder
Taste	Sour	Bitter	Sweet	Pungent	Salty
Smell	Goatish	Burning	Fragrant	Rank	Putrid
Liquid	Tears	Sweat	Saliva	Mucus	Urine
Tissue	Sinews (Muscles)	Blood Vessels	Flesh	Skin/Hair	Bones
Excess Yields	Nails	Coloring	Lips	Body hair	Head Hair
Sensory Organ:	Eyes	Tongue	Mouth	Nose	Ears
Commands	Sight	Words	Taste	Smell	Hearing
Sound	Shouting	Laughing	Singing	Weeping	Groaning
Emotions: Negative	Anger, rage, depression	Impatience, mood swing, cruelty	Worry, sympathy, obsession, pensiveness, desire	Grief, sadness (anguish)	Fear (anguish)
Positive	Kindness	Joy, honor, respect	Balance, honesty, harmony	Courage, righteousness	Gentleness

pression. This pulse is wiry, especially in the middle position; the tongue has a reddish tinge, and the patient complains of a bitter taste in the mouth. Upon questioning, it seems that he is subject to fits of anger. This patient is suffering from a *wood* imbalance, and, specifically, excess in the *gallbladder.* The *Su Wen* states that "decisions are made by the *gallbladder,*" and in this case, we find there is an excess of decision, rashness and impatience.

In the internal environment, we often see a five-phase reflection of the external: for examples, the relationship between DAMPNESS and the *spleen* or WIND and the *liver.* It is a fact that people with *liver* disharmonies are often sensitive to wind and especially prone to problems in the spring, or that people with *spleen* disharmonies suffer during periods of high humidity. From these simple associations has emerged a whole system of complex correlations, somewhat incredible to the Western mind, but understandable in the context of holistic theory.

We must emphasize that the five phases are not static elements; on the contrary, they are symbols which represent changing qualities of movement and matter. They are often confused with the Greek concept of "four elements." We've spent much time pondering these two systems and have come to the conclusion that they are entirely different models. The Greek system of four elements, like much of Western thought, is a more material concept; it is directly concerned with *matter,* while the five phases are more concerned with the *movement of matter,* or qualities of energy. This is their crucial difference and why they cannot be interchanged.

Today, with our great knowledge of chemistry, with the marvel of the periodic table of elements, we can easily scoff at these ancient holistic systems. One frequently hears the argument that ancient people created these primitive models because they knew nothing of the true constituents of matter. This common attitude erroneously overlooks the inherently comprehensive perspective of holistic systems. The five phases are a holistic model of the cosmos, encompassing man, earth, and heaven. Like all models it has limitations, but it does provide a remarkable system of correspondences based on this idea of "qualities of energy." And if one doubts the simple wisdom of these ancient systems, witness these lines from the Nobel prize winner for the discovery of Vitamin C, Albert Szent-Gyorgyi: ". . . [W]hat drives life is a little electrical current, kept up by sunshine [fire]. Water is at the bottom of nature . . . it is the cradle of life, the mother of life."[8]

The practical value of these five-phase correspondences is complex because it requires great clinical experience to sift the useful from the useless. For instance, the *liver* is associated with spring (growth), with the sour flavor, with tendons, and with the emotion of anger. Clinically, one finds many tendon problems associated with the *liver*, and many patients with anger do have *liver* problems; the experienced Chinese doctor, however, knows how to look beyond these rules. He studies the whole picture and takes into account all the facts.

The Six Energetic Layers

Zhang Zhing Jing, a famous Chinese physician, wrote a medical treatise in the 2nd century A.D., *The Shang-han Lun (Cold Induced Disorders)*, which discusses how cold and other factors can penetrate and effect the body. His theory of the six stages was originally conceived as an explanation for the entry of outside evil energies into the body. The following tables illustrate these layers and indicate their relationship to the classical flow of energy through the body.

As time passed, many doctors noted that while the six stages were clinically accurate for cold-induced disorders, they were not as useful in the diagnosis of heat-induced disorders; hence in the 1600's, a supplement referred to as the "four stages," or "four radicals," was introduced. These four radicals were more specifically addressed to the idea of heat-induced disorders.

The "six energetic layers," like the five phases are useful for classifying various types of symptoms due in part to their interesting relationships with classical energy flow. Of particular note here is the French physician Yves Requena's book *Terrains and Pathol-*

Table 11: The Six Energetic Layers

1) Tai Yang (Great Yang)   + + +   Small Intestine - Bladder

Cold entering (fear of cold or wind; fever; headache; and floating pulse.)

2) Shao Yang (Small Yang)   + +   Triple Warmer - Gall Bladder

Exterior/Interior (alternating) fever and chills; bitter taste; lack of appetite; irritability; nausea.)

3) Yang Ming (Bright Yang)   +   Large Intestine - Stomach

Interior heat (fever; perspiration; fear of heat; thirst; rapid, big pulse.)

4) Tai Yin (Great Yin)   −   Lungs - Spleen

Interior (Full, distended abdomen; lack of thirst; vomiting; no appetite; diarrhea.)

5) Jue Yin (Absolute Yin)   − −   Pericardium - Liver

Miscellaneous (*yin* and *yang* act in complex manners; some areas are hot, some are cold.

6) Shao Yin (Small Yin)   − − −   Heart - Kidneys

Deep Interior (Aversion to cold, cold extremities; no fever; great desire for sleep; minute pulse.)

Table 12: The Four Stages

1 Wei - (evil energy enters the protective *chi* of the body)
fever; headache; coughing; slight thirst; tongue
slightly red; floating, rapid pulse.

2 Chi - (evil energy enters the *chi* of the body)
fever without fear of cold; great thirst; yellow
tongue moss; dark, scanty urine.

3 Ying - (evil energy enters the nutritive *chi* of the body)
scarlet red tongue; irritability; restlessness; thirst
not as great as with Chi stage; thin, rapid pulse.

4 Blood - (Evil energy enters the *blood*—very serious)
high fever, delirium; coma, extreme irritability, skin
rashes, nosebleed, blood in urine, vomiting blood.

ogy in Acupuncture. His book, in brilliant detail, describes how these six energetic layers are each a different type of soil (terrain) with predictable diseases (pathology) that grow upon them. One cannot dispute the clinical validity of these six energetical layers as diagnostic tools.

Chi and Blood Patterns

Of all the patterns we study, *chi* and *blood* syndromes are perhaps the most crucial. It is vitally important that these terms be well understood for they—along with *yin* and *yang*—are the foundations of Chinese energetic diagnosis.

Chi and *blood*, together, are the basis for the body and its energy. *Chi* is light, etheric, and active. It is more *yang* than *blood* and constitutes the range of bioenergetic phenomena. *Blood*, nutritive and *yin*, is a more substantial form of energy, heavier and denser than *chi*. *Blood* nourishes, *chi* moves and activates. But what we are talking about here is not such a simple dichotomy because the Chinese concept of *blood*, with all of its various functions and interrelationships, is far more complicated than its strictly physiological Western counterpart.

Deficient Chi and Deficient Yang

First we will discuss DEFICIENT CHI and its related disharmony, DEFICIENT YANG. Because what we call "bioenergy" is our *chi*, it stands to reason that deficiency of this *chi* would result in symptoms reflecting a lack of energy: tiredness; soft, low voice; and a reluctance to move about.

But what exactly distinguishes DEFICIENT YANG from DEFICIENT CHI? For the most part they share similar symptoms, but a state of DEFICIENT YANG includes signs of coldness in the body with such symptoms as: cold limbs, aversion to cold, the body can't seem to get warm enough, puffy tongue, and slow deep pulse. Because *yang* implies fire (internal heat and metabolism), it is easy to see that a deficiency of *yang* would result in coldness. DEFICIENT YANG patterns are usually more serious than those of DEFICIENT CHI.

Deficient Blood and Deficient Yin

From a Chinese energetic standpoint, *blood* includes the fluids of the body; a deficiency of *blood* therefore reflects a loss of these vital fluids, which can result in symptoms like dry skin, anemia, arthritis, dizziness, weak or numb limbs and vision problems (*blood* nourishes the eyes).[9]

Its related disharmony, DEFICIENT YIN (in direct contrast to DEFICIENT YANG) has signs of heat along with DEFICIENT BLOOD symptoms. Signs of heat include the following symptoms: red cheeks, rapid pulse, nervous agitation, night sweats, afternoon sweats, redness on the tongue (especially the tip).

Just as *yang* implies fire, *yin* implies water. For this reason, it is easy to compare the DEFICIENT YIN syndrome to a car overheating from lack of cooling fluids. When the vital fluids of the body are deficient, the organs can overheat in much the same manner as the car. In Chinese medicine, there are several degrees of internal overheating. DEFICIENT YIN is one of the milder forms

Table 13: Deficient Chi and Blood Symptomotology

DEFICIENT CHI   = Low energy
DEFICIENT YANG   = Low fire (i.e. cold)
DEFICIENT BLOOD   = Low fluids
DEFICIENT YIN   = Low fluids (resulting in overheating)

DEFICIENT CHI SYMPTOMS

general weakness
lethargy
pale bright face
shallow respiration
low, soft voice
little desire to speak
dislike of movement
spontaneous sweating
pale tongue material
empty or weak pulse

DEFICIENT YANG SYMPTOMS

(In addition to
DEFICIENT CHI
symptoms add:)
more severe symptoms
appearance of cold
cold limbs
aversion to cold
copious pale urine
puffy tongue
slow pulse

DEFICIENT BLOOD SYMPTOMS

dizziness
thin
emaciated body
spots in visual field
impaired vision
numb limbs
weak tremor in limbs
dry skin or hair
scanty menses
lusterless, pale face and lips
pale tongue material
thin pulse
anemia
stiff joints

DEFICIENT YIN SYMPTOMS

(In addition to
DEFICIENT BLOOD
symptoms add:)
symptoms are not
necessarily more
severe
appearance of heat
agitated manner
red cheeks
warm palms and soles
night sweats
afternoon fevers
low grade, chronic sore throat
insomnia
red tongue material
rapid and thin pulse

of overheating. Whereas DEFICIENT YANG is considered a more severe condition than DEFICIENT CHI, it is important to realize that the same is not true for DEFICIENT YIN and DEFICIENT BLOOD. They are considered to be at the same level of severity. Table 13 summarizes the four conditions we've just discussed.

The Languages of Disharmonies Continued

Chi and *blood* syndromes come in patterns other than the deficiency syndromes we've just disclosed. We mention them briefly below, along with the other major disharmony patterns not yet discussed. In Chapter Seven we will fully clarify these various energetical imbalances. Chapter Seven is the core of our book where we support our major premise: There are universal laws governing health and disease.

STAGNANT (or constrained) CHI: A common disharmony, since the smooth flow of *chi* is the bottom line in good health. An improper movement or blockage of *chi* results in all types of pain, muscle spasms, lumps that move around, distention and soreness.

STAGNANT (or congealed) BLOOD: When the flow of *blood* is impeded, palpable masses and sharp pain can result, along with such signs as fixed lumps, tumors, endometriosis, and angina.

HOT BLOOD: When blood flows through an organ or area that is overheating, HOT BLOOD is often the result. Possible symptoms of HOT BLOOD include: boils, acne, hives, bloody nose, and blood in sputum. (Some of these symptoms can also involve other patterns).

DAMPNESS AND MUCUS: DAMPNESS is the accumulation of fluids in the tissues and other related syndromes such as edema, moist itchy skin and fatigue. This crucial, often misunderstood, category will be clarified fully in the following chapters, along with its stagnation category, mucus.

INTERNAL WIND: When a fire burns, there is a draft produced above it. In Chinese medical thought, there is a similar draft sometimes produced from overheating organs or wood-phase imbalances. INTERNAL WIND, analogous to its climatic counterpart, produces changeable, moving symptoms, like twitching, spasms, and itching. Wind disharmonies are often linked to *liver* malfunctions.

FULL FIRE (excess condition): This is more severe than the signs of fire produced in DEFICIENT YIN. The body in this case is seriously overheating, as in high fevers, in some types of high blood pressure, or in extreme emotional situations like anger.

EPI (external pernicious influence or evil energy): In Chinese medicine the external weather conditions play an important role in affecting our health. Many acute illnesses are said to be caused by EXTERNAL COLD, HEAT, DAMP, and WIND.

TRAUMA: accidents, injuries, cuts, bruises, et. al.

Speaking the Language— Disharmony Patterns in Action

So far we've taken a good look at Chinese energetical diagnosis. Now we must bring this knowledge of the four exams, twelve meridians, eight principles, five phases, six stages, *chi*, *blood*, and *yin/yang* together to be of clinical value. Because this is an *inductive science*, intuition and empirical knowledge play an important role. The primary intent here is to draw from all of these various areas to form a cohesive picture—the pattern of disharmony. With this in mind, allow us to illustrate a few simple cases.

A patient comes into the clinic complaining of a chronic dry cough. Paradoxically, he is tired yet restless. He can't sleep. His tongue has a reddish tip. His pulse is fast and thready, especially in the *lung* position. His cough produces little mucus and he has a dry wheeze. From these symptoms alone, we see a clear picture of the DEFICIENT YIN pattern. Even more precision is nevertheless possible. Taking into account the obvious *lung* disharmony, we can now further extend this diagnosis to DEFICIENT YIN (or DEFICIENT YIN OF THE LUNGS). To be completely satisfied, the doctor examines the other meridians such as the *kidneys,* which often have a relationship to *lung* problems.

If in the above case the cough were not so dry, the tongue pale and puffy, and the pulse empty, we would change the diagnosis to DEFICIENT LUNG CHI, providing there were no other major symptoms. However, if the *large intestine* were also affected, we might call this a METAL PHASE (*lung* and *large intestine*) DISHARMONY. If the *lung* and *spleen* were involved, we could label it a TAI YANG DISTURBANCE. In this way, the language of disharmonies is spoken.

Clinical experience demonstrates that each organ system has its own specific range of possible disharmonies. For example, the *liver* tends to EXCESS HEAT and STAGNANT CHI syndromes, while the *lungs* lean towards those of DEFICIENT CHI, DEFICIENT YIN, or EXCESS DAMPNESS syndromes. Some categories are extremely rare if not impossible. These would be patterns such as DEFICIENT LIVER YANG or DEFICIENT LUNG BLOOD. In Chapter Seven, these specifics will be further discussed.

Clinically, the determination of disharmony patterns is more complex than our illustrations convey. It is the rare patient who fits precisely into a neat little disharmony package. More commonly, patients present complex multiple patterns such as "DEFICIENT LIVER BLOOD WITH WIND AND DEFICIENT KIDNEY YIN COMPLICATING." The final diagnosis is not the static label we find in Western medicine; it is always liable to change, with all the flexibility inherent in *yin* and *yang.* This concept is of vital importance, since the disharmony pattern simply serves as a guideline for the individualized clinical treatment which will follow.

Chinese Medical Therapeutics

Once the Oriental medical doctor establishes his diagnosis, he must then determine a treatment plan which will restore proper balance. As was previously mentioned, Chinese medicine covers a broad range of therapies known as the "eight branches," of which acupuncture and herbs are the most pertinent to this book. The Chinese system of herbal medicine is the most sophisticated in the world. Not only does it include plants, but also minerals and animal sources. Although very complex, with literally thousands of medicinal substances catalogued, this system is beautiful and simple in its basic principles. Chinese herbal medicine has the potential for making a tremendous impact on the world of medicine.

Herbal Energetics

Chinese medicinal substances are classified according to their activity or energetics, determined by *yin/yang* and the five phases. Thousands of volumes on this system have been produced in the last two thousand years. The most famous are: the *Shang-hun Lun* (discussion of cold-induced disorders) written by Zhang Zhong Jing in 220 A.D.; *Ben-cao-Jing Ji-Zhu* (commentary on the book of herbs by Shen Nung) written by Tao Hong-jing in 536 A.D.; and the famous *Ben-cao Gang Mu* (The Great Materia Medica) written by Li Shi-Zhen in 1578 A.D. Li Shi-Zhen's book took forty-five years to complete and is a monumental tribute to medicine.

The vast Chinese materia medica draws its knowledge from hundreds of years of clinical practice and includes substances from all corners of the natural kingdom, some very strange to our ears. Their use can only be understood from the perspective of Chinese energetics. Their materia medica lists such diverse remedies as gypsum, oyster shells, common garden herbals, cinnamon bark, ginseng, scorpions and bear gall bladders. All these healing substances are currently organized by the same natural principles that govern diagnosis: *yin* and *yang*, eight principles, the five phases, and the six layers.

The ancient Chinese herbalists/naturalists were masters of observation. Each herb or healing substance was studied in its natural state to obtain clues for determining its energetical properties. Each herb was respected and studied with the deepest regard for its individual relationship to the universe. Many questions were asked about the plant: what time of year it blossomed;

what color were its flowers; where it grew; what part of the plant was used. Through this system of comprehensive examination, the Chinese formulated specific laws enabling them to determine the medicinal function of any herb. Even the odor of an herb can be used to determine its energetical nature. For instance, a strong scent is of *yang* polarity, while a sweet scent relates to the *spleen* organ/meridian.

> The origin of any herb is ultimately the forces of *yin* and *yang*. They [*yin* and *yang*] create the entire natural setting in which herbs come into being. They create their amazing variegation of color, form, and scent—vehicles for a prodigious range of active forces, powers, and properties. We can define the nature of herbs firstly in time, by considering their origin, appearance, and development; and secondly, in space, by seeing their inner character and outward appearance.[10]

In Chinese medicine, it is understood that simplicity is the underlying order of the universe and that all things are interconnected. The shape, form, and development of a plant has an inner significance and a relationship to the world around it, all of which can be determined by careful observation. For instance, from a study of the movement of the seasons, it is possible to gain a better understanding of the energetic nature of an herb. (Refer to Table 14.)

Table 14

SEASON	CHARACTERISTIC OF THE SEASON	NATURE OF THE HERB
Spring	Sowing	Rising
Summer	Growing	Floating
Mid-summer	Maturing	Peaking
Fall	Harvesting	Sinking
Winter	Storing	Sunken

Herbs that have a close relationship with one season will share the energetic characteristics of that season. For instance, in a case of vomiting or hiccups—symptoms that reflect rebellious *chi* moving upwards—the doctor will prescribe herbs with sinking or sunken qualities, such as roots or late-blooming plants, to balance the wayward energies. The energetics of herbs can also be determined through color, taste and thermal properties.

The color and particularly the taste of an herb can be quite useful for ascertaining its clinical use. This is done through five-phase correspondences. "Red" and "bitter" relate to the *heart;* "yellow" and "sweet" to the *spleen;* "white" and "pungent" to the *lungs;* "blue" and "salty" to the *kidneys;* "green" and "sour" to the *liver.*

The thermal properties of herbs, similarly important to determining its energetic use, are easy to understand. Everyone has experienced the cooling and heating properties of herbs; think of the difference between sucking on a mentholated candy versus one of cinnamon. These thermal classifications are divided into sub-categories: "cold," "cool," "mild," "warm," and "hot."

Clinical experience, of course, plays a major role in the classification of these herbs, especially in the case of the "messenger" herbs. This is a unique class of herbs which target herbal formulas to specific meridians and organs. This medicinal category affords Chinese herbal remedies a degree of refinement unknown to any other system; merely by changing the messenger in a prescription, it is possible to change its entire function.

All of the criteria listed above are taken into account when determining the clinical use of an herb or prescription. Each quality by itself is not completely reliable for indicating its character. For example, all bitter herbs would not be indiscriminately used for *heart* problems. Instead, the characteristics of each herb are considered in their entirety. Chinese doctors through the ages have been extremely pragmatic and down-to-earth, and much information has been gathered through countless generations of clinical practice. What didn't work was discarded, even if it fit theoretically. Nowadays, biochemical information about herbs is being added to the existing energetical information. In China and Japan, scientific research is examining these herbs in a new light.

Herbal Prescriptions

Chinese herbal medicine is usually administered in teas or pills. Anyone familiar with Chinese herbal pharmacies, common in Chinese neighborhoods throughout America, has seen their intriguing displays of medicinal substances. These substances are mixed in carefully-determined prescriptions (some have been used with only slight variation for centuries). There are strict procedures regarding the collection, handling, and processing of these medicines, just as there are specific laws regarding their medicinal use. Studying these laws, one realizes the wisdom of the science of herbal medicine.

As early as the *Shang-hun Lun,* rules were established governing the interactions possible between two herbs in a formula. These six laws are: mutual enhancement, mutual assistance, mutual dislike, mutual control, mutual destruction, and mutual production of toxicity. They are defined in table 15, along with the four roles and the seven recipes, which we will now discuss.

In addition to these six interactions, there is a specific framework, known as the "four roles," used to guide the practitioner in his formulation of the correct prescription. This is another example of the simplicity and genius of Chinese medicine. In Chinese herbal formulas there are four roles or positions to be filled. The key or main herb in a prescription is referred to as the "emperor." Herbs that support or enhance the emperor are known as "ministers." Herbs that reduce side effects or restrict the action of the formula are called "assistants." Lastly, the "messenger" herb directs the formula to a specific organ or meridian, harmonizing and coordinating the formula. By adjusting the proportions of particular herbs or by varying a formula by just one herb, it is possible to completely alter the energetic use of the formula.

Many herbal prescriptions have evolved from antiquity (adding the great weight of extensive clinical experience). These prescriptions are known for their abilities to harmonize specific energetical imbalances. Prescriptions, just like herbs, are classified according to action and composition. Classically, we call these categories "the seven recipes." They are: odd, even, large, small, slow, emergency, fast, and repeating.

Standard herbal formulas often have colorful names, such as "Three Yellow Calming the Spirit Tea." As the name suggests, this formula would have a calming effect. "Gentian Dispersing the Liver Tea" is a blend that is used to cool DAMP HEAT, which can sometimes be the cause of gall stones or high blood pressure. In this particular formula, the emperor is gentian, the ministers are scutellaria and gardenia, the assistants are rheumania, angelica, and bupleurum, and the messenger is licorice. There are many hundreds, even thousands of these prescriptions, all of them tested over the centuries. The doctor always has the option of altering these formulae according to the specifics of the patient. The practical value of these herbal medicines cannot be overestimated. They can improve health, increase energy, and boost the immune system. They may be used preventatively and for all disease categories, including difficult and chronic disorders.

Table 15

THE SIX INTERACTIONS

1) Mutual enhancement	Two herbs of similar action used to support and enhance each other. (synergistic)
2) Mutual assistance	Milder synergy: a major action supported by a lesser herb with similar action. (supporting)
3) Mutual dislike	An herb which interferes with the action of another herb. (antagonistic)
4) Mutual control	One herb controls the action of another herb. (inhibiting)

5) Mutual destruction	An herb which decreases or eliminates the toxic effect of another. (antidotal)
6) Mutual production of toxicity	Two herbs that produce toxic effects when used together. (opposing)

THE FOUR ROLES

1) Emperor	The key herb(s) in a prescription.
2) Minister	Enhances or supports the emperor.
3) Assistant	Reduces side effects or restricts action of other herbs (regulates or adjusts).
4) Messenger	Directs the herbs into specific meridians (harmonizes and coordinates).

THE SEVEN RECIPES

1) Odd	The prescription contains an odd number of herbs. Odd prescriptions are used to treat *yang* conditions.
2) Even	The prescription contains an even number of herbs. Even prescriptions are used to treat *yin* conditions.
3) Large	These prescriptions contain a large number of herbs which are used for treating acute and chronic conditions simultaneously.
4) Small	These prescriptions contain a small number of herbs. Small prescriptions are used when only a single action is required (has a gentle effect).
5) Slow	These prescriptions are slow acting. They are used for tonifying empty conditions.
6) Fast	These prescriptions are fast acting, mostly used for first-aid (emergency) situations.
7) Repeating	Two herbs are repeated alternately because of their opposing nature; used for treating certain complex conditions.

Acupuncture Energetics

Acupuncture is often used in conjunction with herbal therapy, since both treatments can support and enhance each other. Like herbal medicine, acupuncture is based on natural laws deduced empirically through the ages. In attempting to explain acupuncture energetics, we often use the following analogy: Imagine the body as a bioelectric unit with its own circuits and switches. Acupuncture points are specific *loci* where one can manipulate this bioelectric energy, like an electrical engineer who uses many knobs to fine tune a sophisticated recording. Each point can be stimulated, using a wide range of techniques including: needles, pressure, heat, and electricity.

These manipulation sites are located all over the body. Classically, there are 360 acupuncture points located on fourteen major pathways of energy. But, in modern times, over 2,000 points are known (many of these were located with electrical instruments). Each point has a systematic classification which describes its energetic action. Some points or categories of points have specific actions such as warming, draining, dispersing, or tonifying. For example, Spleen-9 (*Yin ling quan*, "*yin* hill spring") and Conception Vessel-9 (*Shui fen*, "divided waters") are both known to exert a diuretic action on the body. The Chinese say that these two points "move dampness," a use that is poetically reflected in their names. The action of the two points can easily be verified in the clinic. With a detailed understanding of the action of acupuncture points, the skillful doctor can reestablish harmony in the body/mind. Some points regulate what the Chinese call "the spirit," meaning they can affect the mental/emotional state of a patient as well as the physical condition. This is certainly an intriguing area of acupuncture energetics. Acupuncture, like herbal medicine, has been shown to exert a beneficial influence on many psychological disorders.

Let us give a few simple examples of how an Oriental medical doctor uses his knowledge to restore health. For instance, a patient might manifest the symptoms of acute overheating (what we in the West would call a "flu" or "fever"): flushed face, pound-ing headache, red tongue, and fast pulse. It is only a matter of common sense that to harmonize this condition, we must cool the patient—rid the heat and build the *yin*. Using acupuncture, one might choose points that are known for their cooling action, such as Liver-2, Stomach-43, and Lung-10, depending on the organs involved. Alternatively or in combination with this treatment, an herbalist would select cooling herbs, possibly *zhi zhi* (*Fructuls gardeniae jasminoides*), *lu gen* (*Rhizoma phragmitis communis*), or *shi gao* (*gypsum, calcium sulfate*).

Another person with a "flu" might have symptoms indicating overcooling: pale and shivering; poor circulation; slow pulse; pale tongue; and great sensitivity to cold. This patient would receive a warming treatment using points such as Conception Vessel-4 and Stomach-36. Additionally, these points would most likely be heated by warming a needle with a pleasant form of heat therapy called "moxabustion" (moxa is an herb rolled up like a cigar and burned like punk). Warming herbs might also be given in the form of a hot tea. Treatments are generally given in a series, depending upon the severity of the condition.

In addition to treatment with acupuncture or herbs, the physi-cian might also recommend a change in diet, special exercise, or changes in lifestyle. While many Chinese physicians are proficient in either acupuncture or herbs, it is the wise physician who uses both. Speaking on this subject, the great physician, Sun Su Mo (560 A.D.) stated emphatically, "Those who [only] apply acupunc-ture or herbs are not brilliant physicians. A brilliant doctor masters both acupuncture and herbal medicine."[11] Together, acupunc-ture and herbs work synergistically, providing a superior form of treatment.

Regardless of the treatment modality selected, the best physi-cians always individualize their treatments. Chu Tan Chi (1282–1385) advocated that physicians prescribe herbs carefully, as if weighing a balance. It was Chu who taught that the doctor should add or subtract from traditional formulae according to the in-dividual situuation.[12] Following this tradition, Chen Hsiu Yuan

(1752–1823 A.D.), author of many lay medical books, would sometimes take up to half a day diagnosing and preparing an herbal prescription. Consequently, his reputation was known far and wide, and he was often brought in to cure difficult cases abandoned by lesser doctors.[13]

In this and the previous chapter, we have undertaken the difficult task of explaining in straightforward terms the vast complexity of Chinese medicine without overwhelming the reader or over-simplifying the subject. Our hope is that we have done justice to this challenging assignment. We have looked at Chinese medicine from an historical and modern perspective, detailed its underlying concept of *chi* and examined its philosophy, diagnostics and language. If we have left you thirsty for more, then our job was well done, and we refer you to our ample bibliography.

6

Homeopathy and Acupuncture in Practice

"Those who test homeopathy and make the experiment, do not escape. Over and over again doctors have studied homeopathy, or have been commissioned to look into it, in order to expose it—only to become its most enthusiastic adherents and exponents.

I suppose not one of us has approached homeopathy otherwise than with doubt and mistrust; but facts have been too strong for skepticism."

Sir John Weir, MD, KCVO, MB[1]

This quote from the former physician to Great Britain's royal family, Sir John Weir, is as true for Chinese medicine as it is for homeopathy. When one first begins the practice of these subtle healing arts, the head is filled with a spectrum of skepticism, insecurity, and wonderment. Does this technique really work? Have I done it properly? Am I really doing anything? Then, inevitably, comes the first remarkable case. The patient's healing response is quite dramatic and only accountable to the little white pills you administered, or to the precisely inserted needles. The novice practitioner is often just as surprised as the patient, and certainly equally pleased. After all the long hours studying a tenuous theory, plodding along on faith and hearsay, achievement is finally realized. Predictably, the excited practitioner attempts to maintain his veneer of authority while his thoughts are wildly proclaiming, "This stuff works—it really does work!" How rewarding it is to spend one's life witnessing these powerful yet gentle healing arts in action.

We, the authors, entered this absorbing field of energy medicine after personally experiencing its efficacy. Louis, at twenty-five, was in the hospital preparing to sacrifice his overworked gall bladder when a friend convinced him to leave immediately and see an acupuncturist instead. Imagine the sight of a tall, determined individual stealing away from the hospital in the middle of the night wearing only a gown! Louis never returned for that operation. His experience with acupuncture literally changed the entire direction of his life. His diet changed, his attitude changed, and most important, his career changed. Now, years later, his gall bladder is functioning better than ever.

Clark, on the other hand, began his study of acupuncture strictly from an academic view. His interest in Chinese philosophy led him to enroll in an acupuncture course. With his collegiate background in science, it is small wonder that he only considered it an interesting example of "primitive folk medicine." During this period of his life, he suffered from a bone spur which gave rise to a chronic sprained ankle. In view of the meager medical approaches to solving this problem, he decided on a whim to try acupuncture. Much to his amazement, the acupuncture treatments cured not only this problem, but eventually his chronic asthma.

It was these direct experiences that intrigued and inspired us in our desire to help others as we had been helped. Even so, both of us entered the study of Chinese medicine filled with plenty of healthy skepticism, which soon faded into the inner knowledge of clinical experience. The same direct experience has led many of our associates to their careers. We suspect that personal experience has stimulated the current profusion of health care professionals who have turned to these safe and effective methods of healing. Indeed, we are witnessing a medical revolution, as holistic medicine takes its rightful place in Western culture.

The purpose of this chapter is to bring to life these medicines we've been discussing. We have carefully searched for cases that are clear, concise and interesting, and which convey the essential flavor and character of both systems. The cases are divided into two sections: one, for homeopathy; the other, for Chinese medicine. Each is prefaced by an introduction to its own particular methodology.

Before beginning these sections, it is important to understand clearly the essential differences in philosophy between conventional medicine and its bioenergetic counterpart. In conventional medicine (the modern biochemical model), diagnosis and treatment resemble war; practitioners speak heroically of the "war on cancer," of "looking for the magic bullet," or of "combating disease." It is a well-known fact that conventional medicine works best when it is able to focus on a specific target and destroy it. This target, the basis of modern medicine, is a specific pathogenic factor, be it a bacteria, virus, cancer, or organ malfunction. The pathogenic factor becomes the enemy, and subsequent therapy is designed to kill, remove, or otherwise dispose of it, usually with drugs or surgical procedures as its fundamental ammunition. Mainstream medicine is based on a mechanistic concept of the body as an inert chemical laboratory where illness is treated by administering chemicals, repairing broken parts, or replacing worn out ones. Conventional medicine typically fails when a precise etiology cannot be found.[2]

In direct contrast, the language of the bioenergetic model is filled with more peaceful terms: "harmony," "resonance," "nurturing," "balancing," and "building." Bioenergetic medicine is a holistic approach that works in conjunction with the natural recuperative powers of the body. It views disease as an energetical concept. These *gestalt* concepts, we reiterate, are termed "patterns of disharmony" in Chinese medicine, and "remedy pictures" in homeopathy. It is the premise of this book that the similarities between these two concepts is no mere coincidence; they both reflect an understanding of universal truth.

Although they derive from very different histories, and draw from distinct bodies of literature, homeopathy and acupuncture share striking similarities. Both systems view the body as a whole and study the relationship of symptoms as patterns, rather than isolated problems. In our busy practice, we have seen patients with multiple symptoms who have been shuffled from specialist to specialist without result, only to respond dramatically to holistic

therapy. It is unfortunate that the majority of such people are totally unaware of the preventative aspects of bioenergetic medicine.
With these medicines it is possible to treat disharmonies while they
are still energy disturbances, before they reach the stage of tissue
pathology that Western medicine treats. Thus the person who seeks
medical attention for fatigue, headaches, or other vague symptoms, where the MD cannot find anything wrong, will often find
that he responds well to bioenergetic medicine; there is no need
to wait for an energetical disorder to develop into a pathological
tissue disorder to benefit from such treatment.

Nevertheless, we should emphasize that bioenergetic medicine
doesn't exclude biochemical medicine. A true holistic doctor uses
laboratory reports and the full complement of Western medical
procedures to evaluate patients. In our practice, we work directly
with medical doctors. When it is warranted, we refer patients to
specialists and surgeons; the vast majority of our patients, however, come to us after conventional medicine has failed.

In taking a person's case history, the holistic doctor devotes
more time and attention to understanding "the whole picture" than
does his allopathic counterpart. Patients respond well to the sympathetic interest shown towards all of their problems, and are often
amazed at the depth of the interview and the interest of the holistic
practitioner in details usually overlooked or ignored by conventional doctors. It is a comfort to realize that the doctor's interest
goes beyond their chief complaint; it is his intention to help with
the minor problems as well, because bioenergetic therapies evoke
the body as a whole to heal. Indeed, in the clinic we sometimes
hear patients saluting us for the cure of a problem they had never
even mentioned. We often joke about those strange "side effects"
of bioenergetic medicine.

Observing this type of physician at work, one cannot help
but be struck by the detail and precision with which the case is
approached. This type of medicine involves the detailed study of
each individual. How or why is this person unique? What is it
about this set of symptoms that is unusual or follows a particular
pattern? Because of the necessity for this type of detail, holistic

casetaking is not easy to learn; it is a complex and lengthy process at which one excels only after years of clinical experience, but the degree of personal contact, and the resultant healing and growth from these interactions, make the mastery of this art well worth the effort.

Homeopathic Casetaking

"The physician's degree of success in obtaining the proper symptom picture lies in his skill and patience. We cannot rush these patients through. We must be good listeners. Get the patient to talking, and tactfully keep him talking about the symptoms rather than wandering far afield. Then cultivate your powers of listening and give your powers of observation full sway to form the complete picture of the little details and habits of your patient. It has been said that criminal lawyers should be medical men; it is eminently necessary, however, that homeopathic physicians be past masters of the art of cross examination; and the observance of the patient's every movement and expression whould be a matter of record.
Herbert Roberts, MD[3]

The homeopathic doctor is perhaps the most painstaking of all medical practioners when it comes to this fine art of casetaking. Dr. Robert's quote alludes to the detail necessary in proper homeopathic casetaking. This chapter can scarcely scratch the surface of this important subject. We suggest that the interested reader refer to our bibliography for further studies in this fascinating field.

The complex field of "chronic prescribing" (what is commonly referred to as "constitutional treatment') is the main focus of this introductory discussion on homeopathic casetaking. "Acute prescribing" for colds, flus, and the like is far simpler but still holds to the basic tenets of individualization discussed here.

From the homeopathic viewpoint, it is especially important to allow the patient to express his history with as much freedom and spontaneity as possible. The practitioner must cultivate the ability to elicit this vital information with as little prompting as necessary. A simple "yes, and what else?" will often yield a wealth of information. When the patient expresses symptoms in his own words with no prompting, these symptoms receive the most weight in remedy selection. It is not until the patient runs out of words that the practitioner completes the history with various questions. We've noticed many times that after the patient claims to be through, careful interrogation elicits yet more vital information. It is of course helpful to know the conventional medical diagnosis of the patient. While this information is sometimes of little importance in remedy selection, it is quite valuable in terms of prognosis and other evaluations concerning the case. Also of great importance in casetaking is a detailed personal and family medical history, all of which might provide valuable clues to the background of the patient's condition.

After the case is taken, a process sometimes requiring one hour or more, the homeopath's work is far from done. Now begins the challenging task of evaluating this mass of symptoms, and proceeding with the remedy selection. This task is accomplished by a careful, systematic weighing and ordering of the totality of symptoms from a case. There are different styles of casetaking, different ways of evaluating symptoms; as an illustration, we will describe one basic approach to casetaking with which we are familiar.

First and foremost, it is essential that the homeopath understand the relationship of each symptom to the trinity of body, emotions, and mind, delineated in most texts as "physicals," "emotionals," and "mentals." Mental symptoms represent the deepest disturbances possible on a total body level, and therefore these symptoms generally receive the most weight in diagnosis. Physicals, involving a lesser degree of importance, consequently receive the least weight. (Of course the intensity or seriousness of a physical can make it quite critical to diagnosis and treatment.) Below, we will discuss each of these in order of importance.

1. MENTALS. Mental symptoms reflect imbalances in a person's mental state; these imbalances can generate deep disturbances

in a person's psyche. Mentals include delusions, paranoia, and forgetfulness—in fact, any deviant behavior affecting clarity, coherence, creativity, or reasoning.

2. EMOTIONALS. Emotional symptoms indicate an imbalance in a person's emotional state: anguish, sadness, apathy, fear, jealousy, and the full range of emotional states.

3. PHYSICALS. Physical symptoms relate to specific tissue problems: liver, bone, brain, muscle, and so on. Examples include muscle spasms, gallstones, arteriosclerosis, and bonespurs.

Next, the homeopath will typically classify symptoms into four broad categories. These categories are: "common," "particular," "general," and "peculiar." Common symptoms are the least valuable to the homeopath, while general and peculiar symptoms tend to be of greatest value.

1. COMMON. Common symptoms are normal to the expression of the disease. For instance, a runny nose would be expected with a cold, diarrhea is usual with intestinal flu, and painful joints are common to arthritis. These types of symptoms are expected during the course of a particular disease and consequently of little value in selecting a remedy.

2. PARTICULAR. Particular symptoms originate from specific areas of the body. They are localized symptoms, very similar to physicals, that include stomach pain, swollen joints, plantar's warts and hemorrhoids. In addition, symptoms that predominate on one side of the body (e.g., left- or right-sided symptoms) are classified as particular.

3. GENERAL. General symptoms describe sensations of the whole body and cannot be localized. Examples would be fatigue, sensitivity to cold weather, or whole-body aches. Descriptions of these symptoms by a patient are usually prefaced with statements such as "I feel," or, "I am." Even though the term "general" is slightly misleading, these symptoms are actually invaluable to remedy selection because they pertain to the body as a whole.

4. PECULIAR. Peculiar symptoms are the strange, rare and un-

usual symptoms that truly individualize a case. The homeopath is delighted when a patient freely offers this kind of distinctive symptom. Peculiar symptoms fall into three types:
1) atypical (of the disease syndrome); 2) "sensations as if . . . .";
and 3) the unusual. A few examples of the atypical type include: painless joints with arthritis; no thirst with high fever;
or slow pulse with elevated temperature. Another type of peculiar symptom which may be described by a patient is prefaced with some version of the phrase, "sensation *as if*. . . ."
For example: "I have a strong sensation *as if* something were
alive in my abdomen"; or, " . . . *as if* the limb were made
of glass and could break easily." Unusual symptoms, the last
type, are just that—unusual. A few of the multitude of possible unusual symptoms are: hatred of human voices; a pain
in the heart when urinating; or a recession of the stool after
it has been partially expelled. These peculiar symptoms can
make remedy selection easier, and are invaluable in the decision to employ rarely-used medicines. But do keep in mind
that we don't prescribe on the basis of a single symptom; we
prescibe on the basis of patterns of symptoms.

In addition to the types of symptoms we've just discussed,
there are other key symptom categories. These are "modalities,"
"sensations," "objectives," "sex" and "sleep."

1. MODALITIES. Modalities are direct modifiers of symptoms,
   and one of the most useful tools available to the homeopath.
   They are the circumstances that affect symptoms. Usually,
   these factors either improve ("ameliorate") or make the symptom worse ("aggravate"). Modalities are diverse and they can
   relate to the time of day, temperature, weather, pressure,
   eating, habits and motion, as well as the various factors that
   exacerbate or relieve symptoms. Illustrations of modalities
   are expressed by: patients who complain that they feel worse
   on humid days (weather); that they feel worse in the afternoon (time of day); or explain that their pain is better after
   getting up and moving around (motion).

2. SENSATIONS. Sensations are descriptions of how various symptoms feel or are perceived by the patient. A few examples of sensations are burning, throbbing, thirsty, and itchy. These clues can be crucial in remedy selection.

3. OBJECTIVES. Objectives or empirical symptoms include the doctor's observations of the patient. These symptoms include such details as facial coloring, restlessness and odors. This type of symptom can also be described by the patient in his session with the doctor, usually in direct response to questions such as: "What color are your stools?"; "Describe your mucus"; and "How does this tension manifest itself?"

4. SEX. Sexual symptoms are matters that pertain specifically to sex, such as frigidity, impotence, or excesses. Sexual concerns have a strong impact on the total health picture of an individual.

5. SLEEP. These are the symptoms that relate directly to sleep: dreams, insomnia, narcolepsy and nightmares.

There are a few other ways in which a homeopath might analyze a symptom. Is the symptom recent or old, chronic or acute? How did it evolve? With what intensity is it described? For example, if a patient casually mentions that he likes to sleep with his window open, it is not as important as when he states emphatically, "Doctor, I simply cannot sleep without fresh air in my room!" The symptom becomes even more significant when qualified with a statement such as, "I really don't understand this fresh air business; I never had this problem last year." Also, the homeopath might find the causative factor of a symptom useful in treatment. All of the various classifications of symptoms enable the doctor to form a clear pattern of the totality and thus prescribe the correct remedy—the simillimum.

To select this simillimum, the homeopath uses two basic tools, the materia medica and the repertory. Classic standards in the field include Boericke's *Pocket Manual of Materia Medica* and Kent's *Repertory*; others are listed in our bibliography.

The materia medica is the mainstay of any viable medical

practice. The homeopathic materia medica, an alphabetical index of the remedies, derives its information from three primary sources: (1) provings (pathogenic); (2) those symptoms derived from reports of poisonings, overexposure, and overdosing (toxicological); and (3) symptoms alleviated through clinical use. In addition, materia medicas contain other useful information about topics such as cross-referencing, modalities, antidotes, and the like.

Imagine attempting to select a single remedy from a materia medica. Even the smallest materia medica contains a hundred or more remedies, some with only subtle differences between them. The use of such a text would be a nightmare without the useful repertory. The repertory is an index to the remedies listed according to symptoms, compiled from the same sources used for the materia medica. Each repertory has its own system of organizing these symptoms, usually according to physical location with separate sections on mental and general symptoms. A few repertories are alphabetical; however, these systems are not commonly used.

It is the function of the repertory to organize this mass of symptoms from all the various provings into a comprehensive index which allows the homeopath to choose the appropriate remedy. When the homeopath utilizes the repertory, it is with the hope that he will clearly see one remedy; however, this is not always the case. More often he is only able to narrow the selection to a few good choices. This is where the materia medica proves its worth. The homeopath uses the materia medica to confirm his selection or to make the final selection from several remedies. If the homeopath has indeed selected the simillimum, the patient will soon be restored to health.

To illustrate how this process works, we present a hypothetical case and analyze it with Kent's *Repertory*.[4] We use, for this example, a patient who complains of lumbar (low back) pain. It should be obvious that lower back pain is not a mental or emotional symptom but a *physical* symptom. Every reader can surely recall at least one person with this common malady; it is exactly this high rate of occurence that also makes this symptom quite plainly a *common* symptom.

Because we can localize this symptom—the pain is in his back—it is possible also to classify this symptom as a *particular* symptom. Looking on page 905 of Kent's book we see over 200 remedies listed with lower back pain as part of their overall symptom picture. This common and particular symptom is simply not specific enough for remedy selection.

If we allow the patient to continue, remembering to let him freely express his story, we will usually discover more relevant symptoms. For instance, he offers, "I feel worse outside in the wind." Now we are getting somewhere; *general* symptoms are often very useful. In Kent's on page 1422 we find this indication listed with fifty-four remedies—better, but hardly allowing more than a wild guess to the simillimum. However, the patient also innocently volunteers that, as strange as it seeems, his back pain not only burns at night but also moves up the spine between his shoulder blades. This is exactly the type of symptom we were hoping to hear—a *peculiar* symptom—one that makes this person's back pain unique. Turning to page 921, we see under "pain, burning," this symptom with five remedies. In the same section, we see that there are three remedies under burning lumbar pain at night. One of these remedies is *Phosphorus*, the only remedy repeated under all the above indications. Upon further examination, this patient reveals other definitive *Phosphorus* symptoms. *Phosphorus* is a well-known, deep-acting constitutional remedy. (Constitutional remedies are those that provide deep relief from a wide range of symptoms and illnesses.)

Of course, in a real case many other symptoms would also be examined through the repertory. If we have indeed found the simillimum then it will heal the back pain as well as many other complaints not mentioned. It is wise to keep in mind that this example demonstrates the various classes of symptoms, but that in real practice all the symptoms in a pattern are important, for they all comprise the picture. Remember, it is the little brush strokes that fill in the details. Homeopathic prescribing is not based simply upon finding peculiar symptoms, but on finding patterns of symptoms and matching these to a remedy. After finding the correct remedy, the homeopath must also determine the potency and how often it must be repeated. This is a tricky area that requires much experience and training.

Following the Case

After the initial prescription in a chronic case, the physician must monitor the patient, who will be rescheduled for evaluation in a few weeks. It is the rare patient who is cured after one visit. Acute prescribing is less complex and can often be dealt with in one or two visits. Managing the follow-up is one of the most challenging and difficult responsibilities that the physician faces, and proper handling of the follow-up is essential for cure. It is the true test of the homeopath's skill and requires the utmost talent and training. During the follow-up, timing is essential. It is a difficult task to know the proper time to change the remedy or its potency, or simply to leave things alone. These decisions can be crucial to the outcome of the therapy, and the cardinal rule is to give no more medicine until the previous one has ceased to act.

Homeopathy requires a high degree of rational and intuitive thought processes working in harmony. The ability to integrate these thought processes produces a rare breed of great physician, practicing an exacting discipline requiring much time, patience, and careful observation. Like good detectives, the people who dedicate their lives to its mastery find pure delight in the detail. At each visit, the homeopath carefully reviews all symptoms, noting the ones that have changed and those that have not. From this careful and thorough analysis, it is possible to determine the exact time to alter or change the remedy. It is in this manner that the homeopath is able to regulate the patient's health pattern and effect a cure.

Homeopathic Cases

To make the practice of homeopathy more vivid for the reader, we present four carefully-chosen cases, representing the wide and diverse range of this holistic science. These cases are from prominent homeopaths of the last century, so they may seem "old-fashioned." For practical reasons we have selected cases relatively free from medial jargon.

Case I

The first case selected is from the casebook of one of the great masters of homeopathy, an American doctor, James Tyler Kent. Kent was a prolific writer and educator, as well as an outstanding clinician. This particular case clearly demonstrates how an adept homeopath differentiates between two similar remedies— *Murec purpurea*, the purple fish, and *Sepia*, a remedy made from the ink sack of a squid. Notice the way this case reads like a detective story:

Pain in Abdomen or Suspected Tumor

On *Murex Pur:* Mrs. K., aged 40, a midwife. She complained of the abdomen; she believed she had a tumor. Severe knife-cutting pain in the region of uterus running up to left breast; pains undefined, running up and through pelvis, worse lying down, aching up and through the uterine region as if the uterus would escape. Empty, "all-gone" feeling in the stomach. Greenish-yellow, leucorrhoea, with itching in labia and mons veneris; intense sexual desire. The os uteri was said to be ulcerated and eroded, and it was sensitive to the touch. The contact of the finger with cervix brought on the sharp pain that she described as running to the left mamma. The uterus was enlarged and undurated. She had been the mother of several children; had had several abortions, and was accustomed to hard work. She had been treated locally by a specialist of acknowledged ability, and she had taken many remedies of his selection as well as from her own medicine case, all very low [potency]. Her catmenia quite normal.

To take up the important and guiding features of this case we must compare several remedies, but principally *Murex* and *Sepia*.

The cutting pain in the uterus has been found under *Curare*, *Murex* and *Sepia*, but *Murex* is the only one producing a cutting pain in the uterus going to the left breast.

The "all-gone" empty feeling in the stomach is characteristic of *Murex, Phos.* and *Sepia.*

Throbbing in the uterus, belongs only to *Murex.* The dragging down is common to both *Murex* and *Sepia,* but the sexual teasing only to *Murex.* Both have a yellowish-green leucorrhoea. Pain in sacrum is common to *Murex, Sepia* and many others. "Enlargement of bowels" is found in Allen [a well known repertory] under *Murex* . . . The pains in *Murex* go upward and through, worse while lying down. In *Sepia* the patient is better lying down, and the pains go around.

Murex 200c, one dose was given. She was much worse for several days. Then improvement went on for two weeks. The remedy was again repeated. One year later she complained of a return of her symptoms. One dose was followed by relief, since which time she has made no complaint, but praises the individualizing method.[5]

Case II

Our second case we take from another well-known American homeopath of the late 1900's, E. B. Nash. Although this case is short—a mere paragraph—it illustrates something of vast importance to homeopathic practice: One prescribes on the basis of patterns, not of disease entities!

In his book, *Leaders in Homeopathy Therapeutics,* Nash recounts:

> I once had three cases of intermittent fever in one family, living in the same house and exposed to the same influences. Quinine failed to cure any of them, and a different remedy, as indicated by the symptoms according to the homeopathic law of cure, was required for each case and promptly cured it. The respective remedies were *Eupatorium perfoliatum, Ignatia* and *Capsicum.* Now any good homeopath can tell you the leading symptoms for all three remedies. That is science.[6]

A curious fact about homeopathy is that it is possible for two people with the same Western diagnosis to be given totally different remedies, while two people with totally different diagnoses might be given the same remedy.

Case III

This case from the files of Dr. Carroll Dunham is a fine example of the wisdom of natural medicines versus suppressive therapies. The homeopathic preparation used in this case is *Mezerum 30 C*, which is derived from the spurge olive, *Daphne mezereum*.

Suppressed Itch: A youth 17, deaf since four, and incapacitated thereby secludes himself and broods over his trouble. Membranes thickened. At the age of three he had eruption of thick whitish scabs, hard almost horny, covering the whole scalp. There were fissures through which exuded on pressure a thick yellowish pus, often very offensive. Much itching and disposition to tear off the scabs with the fingernails, aggravated at night. The treatment (Allopathic) was vigorous; a tar cap was placed on the head and when firmly adherent to the skull was violently torn off, scabs and all, leaving the whole scalp raw. This was painted with a saturated crude solution of Arg Nit. The eruptions did not reappear but from that time the child was deaf. The eruption was the very counterpart of an eruption observed in a proving by Wehle. *Mez. 30* three globules in a powder of sugar milk was given each of these dates—Feb 3, March 1, and September 28, 1857, and January 26, 1858. Improvement set in slowly after the first dose, which was only repeated when the effect of each preceding dose seemed to be exhausted. Finally the hearing was for all practical purposes completely restored.[7]

Case IV

Our next case is a very interesting exchange between two prominent New York City medical doctors, one a homeopath, the other an allopath, who had occasion to discuss a case. This account from the homeopath, Dr. Edmund Carleton, clearly shows the allopathic attitude towards homeopaths as well as the ease with which an accomplished clinician can focus his interrogation to elicit the needed symptoms to complete his picture—all this without the patient even present. In Carleton's conclusion, notice once again the emphasis placed on the need to diagnosis "patterns," not diseases. The failure to understand this basic tenet is a major failing of modern prescribers and scientific investigators, allopathic and homeopathic alike!

One of the best and most favorably known of the [allopathic] physicians of Manhattan, engaged in general practice, came frequently to my office on business of a non-professional character. Our relations were cordial. We never mentioned physic. He was a member of the County Medical Society, fellow of the Academy of Medicine, and otherwise affiliated with the most orthodox associations. One day he tarried after business had been transacted and social amenities observed. Something was in his mind. At last it came out.

"I have a case of gonorrhea that gives me a great deal of trouble. I have done everything for it; but it keeps on; and now the man is in bed with a big orchitis, which gives him more distress than all before it. What would you do for it?"

"Injections?"

"Oh! Yes."

'Cubebs, copaiba, sanmetto and all the rest?"

"Yes, Yes."

"Much pain with micturition?"

"Not great."

"Much discharge?"

"A good deal at first; not much now."

"What consistency and color?"

"Thick and yellow."

"What sort of a looking man is he?"

"Average size, light complexioned, with blue eyes."

"What sort of a disposition has he?"

"Well, I must say, he has been wonderfully good natured."

"How much thirst?"

"I haven't noticed any great thirst."

"Doctor, of course it won't do to promise cure; but I have here a medicine that would, in all probability, cure your patient."

"What is it?"

"That which you would not consider medicine."

"Now I protest. That isn't fair. I am not bigoted. If you say the medicine will cure, let me have it. I will give it as you direct."

"Well here it is" (handing a vial of *Pulsatilla*, two hundredth, in pellets, to him), "give four pellets every two hours until improvement is noted, and then add an hour to every following interval. There must be no other medicine used, locally or constitutionally. When it cures the entire case, let me know, and I will tell the name of the medicine."

Months slipped by before we saw each other again. Our business meanwhile had been transacted in a perfunctory manner, through the mails. I well knew the reason for his absence. Not a word as to medicine passed between us when next we met. The following time, seeing an opening, I said:

"Doctor, did your patient get well?"

"Oh! Yes; it was time for him to get well, after all the medicine he had taken."

My neighbor looked at his watch, and hastened away to meet an appointment. He could not forgive the cure. Fortunately he never learned the name of the successful medicine.

Why did I give *Pulsatilla*? Because of mild disposition; thirstlessness; nearly painless micturition; profuse, thick, yellow discharge; orchitis; for neither of these indications singly but for all combined. It will not cure a case dissimilar to these indications.[8]

Oriental Casetaking

"That I am . . .
paving the way for symptomatic purging and cleansing—
is apparent long before a symptom manifests overtly:

> marking of my irises;
> color and hue of my complexion and aura;
> my hungers and cravings;
> the words I speak, my tone of voice;
> lines and wrinkles of distress on my extremities;
> my choice of activities and entertainment;
> the tenderness of various acupoints;
> sores or blemishes on specific parts of my skin;
> the smell and sounds I emit;
> my responses to various stimuli;
> pain around or within afflicted organs . . ."[9]
> > *The Tao of Health*
> > Michael Blate

The Oriental physician interviews his patients with a simple yet incisive style. The above quote exemplifies the inherent beauty and grace which is the foundation of Chinese medicine. The OMD, as you will remember, utilizes a particular form of interrogation referred to as "the four examinations" (looking, listening, asking and touching). The OMD is even more acutely aware than the homeopath of his own senses during the examination process. During the interview he relies on the totality of his senses, maintaining a well-focused line of questioning and integration of this sensory input. All observation are made from a mind firmly entrenched in Chinese medical philosophy. Is it *yin* or *yang*, outside or inside, hot or cold, excess or deficient? Does it pertain to any of the five phases—*water, fire, earth, wood,* or *metal*?

In a typical interview, when the doctor queries, "Yes, why do you come to see me?" the patient begins relating his story, not realizing how much the doctor already knows of his case. The patient's robust, red face; his curt and abrupt manner; and his obvious propensity for tension have already portrayed a picture of LIVER YANG IN EXCESS. As the doctor listens patiently to the story, it reveals what is already suspected—insomnia, high blood pressure, headaches and dizziness. The patient is quite surprised by the insight of the doctor's line of questions. "Why yes, I have been losing my temper rather easily. I really feel like I'm going to explode at any moment." In this fashion, the doctor is able to guide the patient to relate his medical history. The doctor fills in the gaps of the history with questions regarding diet, exercise, lifestyle, and so on. In conclusion, he takes the pulse and looks at the tongue, which confirm his original diagnosis.

After the consultation, the patient receives an explanation of his energetical disharmony as well as a treatment plan. The actual treatment course can have wide variations, but a realistic series of treatments can be spaced anywhere from three times a week to once every other week for eight to sixteen treatments. During the course of treatment the doctor might offer advice concerning diet, exercise, herbal prescriptions, massage, or some other type of appropriate change. Most people find the acupuncture treatments painless and relaxing. We can't even begin to count the number of patients who have actually fallen asleep during treatment for insomnia or anxiety. Children usually respond well to treatment, and many actually enjoy it, especially as they experience the sense of well-being it offers.

Careful evaluation of the symptoms and systematic observation of the patient, with special attention paid to the pulse and tongue, allow the OMD to determine the precise energetical disharmonies from which the patient is suffering. The whole of Chinese medicine is designed around the shrewd observations of these natural laws, and through their wise application the physician can regulate and restore health. The OMD with his eight branches of therapeutics is quite capable of curing as well as preventing disease. In the following cases, please keep in mind that these simple verbal descriptions do not convey the full experience of Chinese diagnosis and treatment.

Chinese Medical Cases

Case I

The oldest school for acupuncture in the United States is the New England School of Acupuncture, our alma mater, founded in 1975 by Dr. James Tin So. Dr. So graduated in 1934 from the College of Scientific Acupuncture, in Canton, China. His principle teacher was Tsan Tien Chi, who was a student of Ching Tan An, a renowned Chinese doctor. Dr. So was not a sophisticated acupuncturist. He was from a peasant background, pragmatic, compassionate, and simple, with years of experience treating in remote locations where no conventional therapy was available. He therefore had the unique opportunity of resorting to acupuncture for such serious diseases as gonorrhea, epileptic seizures and pneumonia. The case we've selected represents the practicality of his methods, as well as giving the readers some insight into his down-to-earth, direct style.

CASE #14 ACUTE BLINDNESS
DATE: Summer, 1956
PLACE: Hong Kong

PATIENT: Daughter of Mr. Lee, who is the secretary of the Hong Kong Herbalist Association.

CAUSES: This patient has a very bad temper and was very easily angered. She also liked to read novels. Every night she would read until very late before sleeping. She did this for several years. She also was married with several children. Her right eye was blind for many years. She continued reading every night by her one good eye.

SYMPTOMS: One day the patient awoke to find that both eyes were blind. She became very frightened. She called her father and told him her condition. Her father knew a number of good doctors. He took her to many famous doctors, eye specialists, but her condition did not improve. This went on for about 10 days. He then brought her to see me.

POINTS: GV 4, Bl 18.

TREATMENT: In the beginning I used the points recommended for general eye disease: Li 4, St 8, GB 15, Bl 1, Bl 2, TW 23, GB 1. The next day she came back but there was no improvement. Then I had her tell me all about her living habits. I understand from her pulse that the *liver* is too strong and the *kidney* is too weak. The *liver* is too strong so that there is not enough *fire in the life door* [KIDNEY YANG]. I also remember from my teachings that GV 4 should be used for blindness along with Bl 18, I determined to use these points. I treated Bl 18 first, stimulating the point bilaterally for 30 seconds. This drew down the overheating from the liver. Then I treated GV 4 with the needle followed by 10 red bean size direct moxa. After this I had her father take her home. The next day she came back with her father. She said "When I woke up this morning, I could see everything." I treated her once more as above, except I used only 5 direct moxa on GV4. After this case, I did see Mr. Lee again on the street. His daughter had no recurrence of this problem.[20]

Case II

Our second case is from the *Web That Has No Weaver*. This book by Ted Kaptchuck, OMD, is one of the best works on Chinese medicine in any language. Dr. Kaptchuck, an American, received his OMD degree from the Macau Institute of Chinese Medicine in 1975 and was also one of our primary teachers.

CLINICAL SKETCH: Some interesting examples come from two studies that explored the efficacy of Chinese medicine in treating the Western medical entity known as systemic lupus erythematosus (SLE), a serious and often fatal autoimmune disease.

Two studies, the first dealing with 120 cases of lupus, the second with 22 cases, both concluded that traditional herbal treatments reduced the mortality rates from lupus more effectively than Western therapy, and that in a high proportion of cases, Chinese medicine is very helpful in treating the disorder.

The first study found that several distinct disharmony patterns arise when diagnosing SLE. Here is a case history from the second study, which emphasized *Kidney* patterns.

One May 23, 1960, a woman, aged thirty-two, came to the hospital complaining that her facial skin, especially her cheeks, seemed to have injuries similar to frostbite. The condition had gradually gotten worse over the previous six months. She also complained of sore joints and back pain, dizziness, palpitations, insomnia, night sweats, and an occasional low fever. She was often thirsty, but had no desire to drink. Since the illness began, her hair had been falling out and her menstrual blood had diminished.

The Chinese examination noted a depleted *spirit*, thinness of the whole body, low voice and dark complexion. Her cheeks had a purple-red rash, the center of which was gray and scaled. Her eyes were sunken and darkish in the sockets; her hair was thin; the tongue moss was thin and white; the tongue material was cracked and bright red; and the pulse was thin and slightly rapid, with the third position especially weak.

Following the Chinese clinical examination, the patient was given a battery of Western medical tests. Some of the lab findings include: white blood cell count 2,400/mm³; red blood count 3.06×10^6/mm³; total protein 8.6 grams percent; platelets 54,000/mm³; sedimentation rate 32 mm/hour (Cutler). An electrocardiogram showed arrhythmia, LE prep negative.

The dizziness, night sweats, heart palpitations, recurring low fevers, cracked and red tongue, and thin and rapid pulse all pointed to DEFICIENT YIN. The backache, the weak third position on the pulse, the darkened eye sockets, and the loss of hair suggested that the Deficiency was in the *Kidneys*. The joint soreness was interpreted as WIND INVADING THE SURFACE MERIDIANS, OBSTRUCTING THE QI AND BLOOD. The rash on the face was thought to be the HEAT OF DEFICIENT YIN AFFECTING THE BLOOD, thus resulting in skin eruptions.

The Chinese physician chose an herbal treatment that combined fourteen herbs to nourish the *Kidney Yin* and *Blood*, cool the *Blood*, and expel *Wind*. The herbs used included *Rehmannia glutinosa*, *Polygonum multiflorum*, and *Paeonia lactiflora*. The patient was given a prescription to be taken daily for eighteen days. When she returned for the next examination, the rash had somewhat subsided. She was given a slightly different prescription. By the time she returned in five days the rash had been very visibly reduced, her appetite had improved, and her joints were less sore. The backache, palpitation, and night sweats were all gone. White blood cell count was 4,500/mm^3, red blood cell count was 3.84 × 10^6/mm^3, and platelets were 98,000/mm^3. The patient continued to show improvement with additional treatment.[11]

Case III

The third case comes from one of the authors, Clark Manning. This case, another portrait of DEFICIENT KIDNEY YIN, was chosen because it demonstrates how Oriental medicine, like homeopathy, treats a *pattern*, not a disease. Here I treat a case of rheumtoid arthritis in much the same fashion as the above case of lupus. I should mention that I've treated many cases of rheumatoid arthritis that were not DEFICIENT KIDNEY YIN and also that not all cases responded as well as this one.

Mrs. O., early forties, suffering from rheumatoid arthritis. Her chief complaints, other than the obvious pain from her deformed knuckles, are insomnia, lower back pains, night urine, dizzy spells, and headaches. She is obviously a nervous person and interrogation uncovers a great deal of anxiety. Further questioning reveals the peculiar symptom—her ears are always hot. And indeed, there is actually a noticeable red tinge to them. Pulse diagnosis indicates a weakness in the KIDNEY YIN position with a tight threadlike overall quality. Her tongue is thin and pointed with a red tip. It quivers somewhat as she extends it for observation. I diagnose her as DEFICIENT KIDNEY YIN and recommend a lengthy series of treatments, explaining that rheumatoid arthritis is very difficult to cure. However, there is an excellent chance because we are catching it so early.

During the course of treatments it was most rewarding to see the gradual changes that developed in this woman. She had a keen sense of humor coupled with a fine optimistic spirit. At first nothing happened, but she continued coming, stating, "The treatments are relaxing enough alone to make them worthwhile." Later she informed me that there was no doubt about it, she was definitely sleeping better and her night urine was diminishing. As time passed, most of her symptoms were improving and by the fourth month her hands were free from pain. She was ecstatic as it became clear that her arthritis was reversing itself. By the end of six months her hands looked normal, with no trace of arthritis, and her ears had lost their redness and heat. It was amusing to listen to her tongue-in-cheek complaints that she now had to wear earmuffs. "I've never worn ear muffs in my life!" she would joke.

Case IV

Our last case, an anecdote from Britain's leading medical journal, *The Lancet*, is most interesting because it graphically illustrates the typical amazement when a conventional Western doctor discovers the efficacy of acupuncture.

The Lancet, June 13, 1981
BACK PAIN AND ACUPUNCTURE
SIR, I was interested in your May 2 editorial on back pain. As a physician who is a regular sufferer from the 'idiopathic type,' I fully sympathise with my similarly-afflicted patients and share with them the painful realization that all conventional treatments are pretty useless. Your editorial did not mention one line of therapy that has been available for thousands of years, well before analgesics, local anaesthetics, and so on, yet continues to be shunned by doctors and medical journals alike-namely, acupuncture. My own personal experience this week has totally changed my view on this unorthodox therapy.

Five days into the throes of acute back pain with increasing muscle spasm and pain and the increasing assumption of a Groucho Marx posture led me, without much optimism, to turn to acupuncture as a last resort. Contrary to my assumption, this was a very painful procedure. I was assured by my therapist that relief would be virtually immediate. To my chagrin I could not leave the couch. The pain was worse, the spasm almost tetanic. Angry doctor intimating dismay to increasingly blushing therapist. Doctor now walking out of surgery like Groucho Marx with kyphosis. Crawls into car, 30 minute drive home. Doctor convinced that he had been 'had'—foul sorcery had been the order of the day. Convential medicine, although useless, must be better than this nonsense. *The Lancet* has been correct not even to mention this dastardly affront to scientific endeavour.

Fuming doctor now blows horn in driveway, wife summoned to help from car. Slow writhing movement to get out of car as painlessly as possible. But something wrong here. Pain almost gone. Look children, daddy is now 6 inches taller than when he left this morning; he can stand straight. Disbelieving doctor, convinced of an artifact, bends forward and back several times as if praying to house. Can move, straighten, walk, hardly any pain. It worked. *The Lancet* had after all made a mistake.

Perhaps millions should be spent researching this therapy which might lead us to save tens of millions on painkillers, muscle relaxants, days off work, hospital beds. Perhaps our editorials could start the ball rolling by at least intimating that throughout the past several thousand years probably more people have derived benefit from this therapy than from any of the 'potions' that your article refers to. Perhaps editorial writers might ask their medical colleagues how many of them have ever availed themselves of acupuncture (but will not admit it publicly). They will be as surprised at the result of this survey as I was that the therapy worked.[12]

[Authors' note on pain: Most people (including children) find acupuncture painless. However, sometimes people in acute pain, especially with *liver* involvement, will find acupuncture extremely painful. This discomfort disappears as the condition improves. There is also a small number of people, not in pain, who find acupuncture painful. These people usually respond very well to treatment.]

In preparing for this chapter we reviewed a large number of interesting cases. Narrowing them to a handful was a difficult but inspiring task. We could not help but notice the dedication, integrity, and compassion of these men, all equal in their desire to help people. And it is clear that each one felt he was doing exactly that—helping people by facilitating the healing process. Those of us lucky enough to be involved in bioenergetic medicines have all witnessed a healing phenomenon that needs to be communicated. This is what impels us each to write.

7

Disharmony Patterns and Remedy Pictures

" . . . to understand anything one must penetrate suffi-
ciently deeply towards this ultimate pattern."
" . . . everything in this universe bears some relation to our
own nature, its needs and potentialities. Every process
mirrors some process in ourselves and evokes some emotion, though we may not be aware of it."
L.L. Whyte (1954)
Scientist and author

Disharmony patterns represent the very heart of this
book. Far from being dull or dry, they are a fascinating and
multifaceted picture of different bioenergetic disorders. To present our major theme, we have chosen fourteen homeopathic remedies. Each remedy is presented from a homeopathic point of view,
then examined from a Chinese medical perspective. In each remedy
one sees that the homeopathic remedy picture corresponds to a
Chinese disharmony pattern, a correlation that illustrates the
universal patterns of disharmony. This correlation does not mean
that these systems are interchangeable, but it does indicate, beyond
doubt, a similar holistic approach to disease and health.

These two medical systems, from completely different cultures, recognize that disease is not just an entity localized in one
part of the body. Disease, or disharmony, first manifests itself in
the bioenergetic field of the body. This field is a holistic phenomenon unifying mind, body, and spirit. In health it is balanced and
resistant, exerting a harmonizing influence over the whole body
and person; in disharmony, imbalances or weaknesses in the field

produce an array of signs and symptoms, often those complaints that impel us to see a doctor.

The headache or muscle spasm itself is not the disease, but the sign of an underlying imbalance. The doctor must, of course, examine the local symptom, but to ensure a fundamental healing, he must observe the whole patient. By "reading" the whole person he can then discern the patient's disharmony pattern. Homeopathic and Chinese doctors read these patterns, but use their respective terminology and methods for diagnosis and treatment. In both systems the intent is the same: to stimulate the healing process and to balance the bioenergy. In the philosophy and methods of these two systems, we discover the essence of holistic medicine. Holistic medicine does not consist of a patchwork of different theories and methods; it is based on the unifying phenomenon. Great philosopher-doctors have recognized this fact since the dawn of civilization.

The homeopathic doctor balances the disharmony pattern by giving the similar remedy, that remedy which most closely matches the totality of the patient's symptoms. We like to use the analogy of the wave form to explain this phenomenon. In health the bioenergetic field is in relative balance and displays an even, regular wave form; in disease this wave form becomes irregular, with deep valleys and high peaks. The remedy, a specific wave form, is viewed as a phase inversion of the irregular pattern and thus cancels it, resulting in balance. Perhaps within this analogy lies the key to the reality of homeopathic provings.

Each remedy, a gestalt, presents the whole picture of the patient's suffering, including physical, emotional and mental symptoms. For example, the remedy *Rhus toxicodendron,* one of several remedies commonly used for arthritic symptoms, has a distinct pattern of physical symptoms. The true distinguishing characteristics of this remedy are not so much the common complaint of stiff and painful joints, but the unique way these symptoms manifest, especially in the case of the modalities.

Modalities are the specific reactions the patient has to circumstances such as weather, time of day, or exercise. In homeopathy and Chinese medicine, modalities are extremely important guidelines in determining the treatment. The modalities for *Rhus tox* are distinctive: The patients' symptoms almost always improve with movement and worsen with damp, cold weather. They like warmth, sun, and heat in any form. Mentally, such patients can be restless and despondent, and all their symptoms are worse during the night. A patient presenting these characteristics along with arthritic symptoms might be given *Rhus tox* by the homeopathic doctor, but only after he has studied the whole case. Homeopathic and Oriental doctors are interested in the unusual and individualistic symptoms—even if they seem unrelated to the presenting problem—because these are often reliable guides to the correct treatment. All the complaints, whether physical, emotional, or describing some unusual sensation, are part of the whole picture and in total create a disharmony pattern.

The Chinese doctor studies the patient to determine imbalances in the energy field and organ systems. As we have discussed, his guidelines are *yin/yang*, the five phases and the twelve meridians. Like the homeopathic physician, he studies the person and his wide range of complaints and reactions, such as his response to climate, particular emotions, and sleep. The disease categories used by Western doctors, useful in studying pathology, do not take into account the individual reactions of people, and often the biochemical doctor will be so intent on local pathology that he ignores the person as a whole. In conventional medicine people complaining of ulcers routinely receive the identical treatment. In holistic medicine these same people would receive an individualized treatment according to the specific characteristics of their condition.

The local symptomatic approach, based on disease categories, can be very valuable in treating such isolated pathological symptoms as acute infectious disease or back pain, but in many instances this approach is superficial, its intent being to eliminate the main symptom while overlooking the person and underlying energetic or psychic factors. In conventional practice this attitude towards strict symptomatic approach is changing. For many years the routine response to fevers was to suppress them with aspirin and other drugs, but in the past few years doctors are realizing that fevers are a useful defense effort to rid the body of harmful bacteria and toxins. If the fever is artificially suppressed by drug therapy, the body is not allowed to complete its natural healing process. It is now common sense to let fevers alone unless they are dangerously high.

Suppressive therapy can have serious consequences, especially when the healing process is cut short by repeated therapy with strong drugs. For over a hundred years homeopaths have claimed that suppressive therapy can drive illness deeper into the body, and that in time this will result in a more serious illness. Skin disorders are often suppressed with cortisone, but often, months or even years later, the same patient suffers from asthma; what was once a skin problem is now a deeper problem in the lungs.

In true holistic medicine such as classical Chinese medicine and homeopathy, the reactions of the whole person are studied. One does not chase symptoms, nor palliate; one avoids suppressive therapy by working with the body and supporting the inherent healing response. The homeopathic response to a simple fever— if it is necessary to treat at all—is to stimulate the body to heal by giving the remedy that will enhance the body's healing process. The doctor's remedies serve as a catalyst for the healing force; he has a deep respect for the healing power of the body, and he tries not to intervene in the natural process. The best way to accomplish this simple and beautiful ideal in healing is to recognize the phenomenon of bioenergy, the unifying influence in the health of the body and spirit. By recognizing the bioenergetic disharmony pattern, the doctor can then catalyze the healing process.

Disharmony Patterns/Remedy Pictures

During the initial research for this book, five years ago, we meticulously studied one hundred and twenty homeopathic remedies, and observed many connections between homeopathy and Chinese medicine. The differences between these systems were quite obvious—for instance, the use of needles versus potentized remedies—but we also saw some startling underlying similarities, such as the parallel use of modalities for differential diagnosis. Increasingly curious, we began to examine these remedies from a Chinese perspective. As we realized the potential of our research, we started to compare the medical philosophies and practices of these two great systems. The most challenging aspect of our research was whittling down the 120 remedies to a select group best depicting the major themes of this book. The fourteen remedies chosen present a vivid picture of homeopathic treatment as well as a broad range of Chinese medical disharmonies. They best represent our theme of disharmony patterns and offer the reader insight into homeopathy and Chinese medicine. But of greatest importance, the reader will gain an understanding of the ageless and universal wisdom of disharmony patterns and how they can be used in a clinical setting.

Before we start this section, we would like to remind the reader that the homeopathic remedy pictures were derived from provings, toxicological reports, and, to a lesser extent, clinical experience. Provings are directed by homeopathic doctors. Healthy volunteers take repeated doses of the potentized remedy until the symptoms of overdose emerge; these symptoms are not only physical—stiff neck, stomach ache, et. al.—but emotional and mental as well. The prover might, for example, develop a frontal headache as well as a bad temper. He might also become extremely sensitive to cold wind. These peculiar symptoms are of extreme importance. The purpose of the proving is to discover the specific effects of a safe, homeopathic dose of a substance; the final picture will indicate its full curative potential. Further information about the curative potential of the remedy can be derived from toxicological reports (medical reports of poisoning). All this information can be substantiated and enhanced by years of clinical experience, and ultimately results in the complete remedy picture.

We present the following fourteen homeopathic remedies in a logical order. Each remedy clearly depicts a different, major Chinese disharmony pattern. The order of these remedies is important because they are arranged according to the development of Chinese energetics.

For each remedy we first give a general description of the substance, including pertinent scientific and medical information, as well as interesting historical facts. We then discuss the homeopathic remedy picture, first by presenting a brief history and description of its preparation, then by discussing the characteristics and keynotes of the remedy. We have culled this data from many homeopathic books, and have attempted to represent fairly the fundamentals of each remedy. Because this book is not a clinical text, we present only major keynotes relevant to understanding the remedy.

In the final section on each remedy we study the homeopathic model from a Chinese medical perspective, demonstrating that each remedy is a clear depiction of a Chinese medical disharmony. Indeed, these homeopathic remedy pictures could be used to teach students about Chinese energetics. Each system gives its own unique name to the universal patterns of disharmony: In homeopathy, each pattern is named for its respective remedy; in Chinese medicine, it is named for an energetical disharmony. Let us give a simple example.

A homeopathic doctor sees a patient with a sharp frontal headache, gastric disturbances from rich food, and an impatient, irritable manner. After taking the complete case the homeopath decides that the patient needs *Nux Vomica,* the remedy which would produce similar symptoms in a healthy person. If this same patient were to visit a Chinese doctor, he might state that the patient is suffering from LIVER ENERGY INVADING THE STOMACH. They have both studied the person carefully. They are both essentially examining the same disharmony pattern, but each gives the pattern a different name. The two treatments, of course, are different from one another, but the objective is the same: to restore harmony with minimum intervention. We find the correlation between these two systems fascinating, a fact that must be pondered for a long time to be truly appreciated.

It should be emphasized that our assessment of homeopathic

remedies from a Chinese perspective is not a precise diagnosis. Our study is not meant to be a rigid classification. We realize that other Chinese doctors will use slightly different terminology and have different opinions; we welcome these. Our intent is simply to explore this idea of disharmony patterns and its role in medicine.

The reader must also bear in mind the difference between the Western and Eastern view of the body. He must temporarily suspend his customary idea of disease categories. The Chinese disharmony patterns are first based on disharmony in the energy of the body. When we say that a patient is suffering from LIVER YANG RISING, this does not mean that the person has a diseased liver. What the Chinese call the *liver* is certainly connected to its anatomical organ, but is broader in function because the Chinese *liver* is simultaneously an organ, a center of energy and a meridian. The Chinese view the body essentially as a map of the flow of vital energy through the various energy centers, each of which has a variety of energetic functions. For example, what is called the *spleen/stomach* is the center that converts food into *chi* and then transports it to different parts of the body. This center includes the diverse organ functions from a Western physiological view, but it also involves a meridian and emotional/mental characteristics. Western medicine looks at the body as an assemblage of organs, each having its own physiological functions; the Chinese did not study anatomy and physiology with such precision. The Western doctors, on the other hand, totally ignore the energetic aspect of living dynamic people, preferring what is called "the mechanistic perspective." Because the Chinese organ/meridian centers are not the same as their Western cousins, we will always italicize them so the reader remembers the distinction. The "*liver*" is not the same as the "liver"!

The patterns of disharmony that we discuss are universal: they hold true for all people of every race throughout the course of history. Historically diseases have altered in certain cases, but the way in which people manifest sickness does not change greatly. In these remedies the reader will see reflections of himself, as well as those of friends and relatives. Many of these remedies have been used since the dawn of history, by ancient Greeks, Indians, monks, Oriental herbalists, and, more recently, by modern physicians. Some of the remedies are exclusively used by homeopaths; these will certainly pique the imagination of the reader.

Remedies are often described as if they were people, because major homeopathic remedies represent types of people. We like to think of these remedies as holographic models of human behavior. Like Plato, Goethe, Paracelsus, and Carl Jung, Samuel Hahnemann intuited the inherent truth of archetypes in matter, but his unique contribution was to apply this knowledge to a system of medicine. Hahnemann found these healing archetypes in the three kingdoms of nature: animal; mineral; and vegetable. Each kingdom offers its own unique gift. Snakes, for example, provide potent venoms—used in many medical systems throughout history—that have been transformed into safe homeopathic remedies. Homeopathy adds a *new* depth to understanding the potential of these healing agents.

Through his extensive provings and clinical experience, Hahnemann came to realize that the major remedies depict clear personality pictures, archetypes of different kinds of behavior. *Nux Vomica*, for instance, is aggressive and impatient; *Pulsatilla*, gentle and timid; *Lachesis* (a snake remdy), volatile and changeable. Each of these remedies has a unique force field that finds a ready resonance in the world of men and women. Edward Whitmont, M.D., who studied with Carl Jung, expounds on this idea of remedies as archetypes:

> Paracelsus postulates gestalts or archtypical patterns which underlie human, as well as extra-human or material phenomena, establishing a complementary, functional relationship between them: Sun (and incidentally gold . . . which is the material manifestation of the Solar principle) corresponds to the heart and its functioning, other substances to other functions.

Whitmont adds:

> Hahnemann . . . fashioned the abstraction of the totality of the drug picture (from the provings). . . . It is the archetypical image according to Goethe's postulate. Jung's concept of arche-

type per se and its visibility as image, patterns of emotion and behavior corresponds to these fields of pure shapes and the visibility in matter. . . . All these concepts add up to the idea of form or gestalt, elements that are more than the sum of the parts, the parts being integrated into an overall pattern by the law of form. This is the angle that Hahnemann intuited in creating what he called . . . the picture or images of remedies as though they were personalities, Miss Pulsatilla, Mr. Sulphur, or Mrs. Sepia.[1]

Chinese medicine and homeopathy recognize these different types but give them different names. When the *Nux Vomica* type becomes excessive in his life style or when his job stresses reach a high level, he begins to display signs of disharmony corresponding to his type. These signs will display a certain pattern, but they will also be unique. *Nux Vomica* will be seen as his constitutional remedy, that which most closely corresponds to the totality of his condition and type. Sometimes, however, he will need other remedies or different forms of treatment. It is this Mr. *Nux Vomica* or Miss *Pulsatilla* that we are going to explore in this following section. These "remedy pictures" or "disharmony patterns" are a window into a completely different approach to medicine, one that is founded on ancient philosophical concepts, and grounded in a practical and scientific approach to healing. There is no reason why these ideas cannot be incorporated into modern biochemical medicine, for both sides will prosper from this union.

These disharmony patterns and remedy pictures make the study and practice of medicine a human science, involving a broad understanding of life and people and incorporating scientific, creative and humanistic concepts. These systems are the antithesis of the specialized modern man, the busy, brain-centered being who knows life only from his specialty. Homeopathy and Chinese medicine require a more universalistic viewpoint; they involve a wide-angle lens, so to speak, not precise tunnel vision. Furthermore, the special challenge for these systems is that this wide-angle lens must also include biochemical facts, just as the biochemical model must become more inclusive. For medicine to be complete, the human being must be seen in relation to the world around him; in the context of people, society, climate and the cosmos; and in relation to the similar cosmos within himself, his inner environment of body, emotions, thoughts and energy.

Aconitum Napellus: Ranunculae

Common *Aconite*, also known as "Wolfsbane" or "Monkshood," is a tall, beautiful, flowering plant that has been used in medicine through the ages. The blossom is a dark violet flower in the shape of a helmet or monk's hood (hence the common name). In former times the whole plant was made into a poison used to dispatch enemies. Its primary alkaloid, aconitine, is a formidable poison that rapidly paralyzes the heart and respiratory centers. The pulse is slowed as well as the respiration, the skin becomes moist and cool, and a profound prostration results in numbing of the lips and mouth. Death from overdose can occur in half an hour to six hours. It is interesting to note that the pharmacological action of aconitine is stimulating and then depressing to the central and peripheral nervous system. *Aconite* is an example of a drug that poisons in large doses but is wonderfully curative in small doses.

Aconite was introduced into modern medicine by Anton von Stoerck in 1762, and admitted into the London Pharmacopoeia in 1788, but presently the drug is rarely used in conventional medicine. It has a long history of use, however, in herbal medicines all over the world, and in the West it was first mentioned in the *Meddygon Myddofai*, published in Wales in the twelfth century.[2] Mrs. M. Grieve, herbalist, claims that *Aconite* is a useful medicine, used carefully in small doses as a local painkiller, diuretic, and diaphoretic.

In China a similar species, *Aconitum Carmichael Detox.*, was used for centuries, long before it was formally recognized in the West. The Chinese pharmacists have developed an ingenious method to lessen its poisonous quality, which involves soaking, drying, steaming, slicing and mixing it with other herbs. *Aconite* is used to expel external cold (for example, colds and flus), to relieve pain caused by cold lodging in the body, and to dispel DAMPNESS due to a deficiency of the *spleen* and *kidney* from shock and collapse. The Chinese call this plant a "warming drug" with the power to expel internal cold.[3] In Western terms, *Aconite* can treat colds, edema, rheumatism and diarrhea, but only according to the individual Chinese indications. The herb would not be prescribed for a disease category but for a person displaying symptoms that specifically indicate the *Aconite* picture. In modern medicine the major alkaloid, aconitine, is employed in treatment because it is the most powerful chemical in the plant; practitioners of herbal and holistic medicine, on the other hand, use the plant itself. The biochemical model requires a specific quantifiable chemical that is targeted for a specific pathological malfunction, while in the holistic model the integrity of the whole is maintained, conserving inherent qualities of the remedy that might not be determined by chemical analysis.

Keynotes and Characteristics

Recognizing the healing potential of *Aconite*, Dr. Hahnemann converted it into one of the most valuable homeopathic remedies, one that is found in every homeopathic first-aid kit. Because of its well-defined symptoms as derived from provings, *Aconite* is one of the main remedies for flus, fevers, and inflammatory states. By introducing *Aconite*, Hahnemann was able to reduce the practice of bloodletting, formerly the major method of reducing fevers in conventional medicine. Some of the primary indications for *Aconite* are:

- Acute fevers that come on suddenly and severely, often after exposure to cold wind. Great fear and anxiety with restlessness and irritation. Symptoms come on so suddenly that the patient fears he is going to die.
- Acute rheumatic pains in the joints after exposure to cold. Intolerable pains. Fever: skin dry and hot, face red and pale alternatively. Thirst for large quantities of water. Loud, rough cough.
- Better: in the open air; after sweating; after rest.
- Worse: in a warm room; in the evening and at night; in dry, cold winds.

These keynotes represent a sample of the symptoms established in provings. The prospective patient must reveal the *Aconite* pattern, not just one or two isolated symptoms.

Chinese Diagnosis

Homeopathic *Aconite* is used to treat what the Chinese call EXTERNAL COLD. The Chinese classify acute diseases such as colds and flus as diseases triggered by external pathogenic factors. The primary climatic factors considered are: cold, wind, damp, heat, and dry (or a mixture: for instance, "cold wind"). Both homeopathy and Chinese medicine recognize the strong effect that environmental conditions have on health.

If we acknowledge that the internal environment can mirror the external one, then we can see how continual exposure to a cold wind would affect a susceptible person. When cold invades the body, the body tries to expel it, the result often being a fever, headache and faster pulse. If the person's vital energy is weak, cold can lodge in the body causing local stagnation and pain, and in certain instances, cold can turn to heat (*yin* turning to *yang*) and the person can display a host of heat signs, as in the case of *Aconite*.

A Chinese text states:

> The vital factors of the human being are closely related to the changes in the weather. The body has to constantly adjust its internal functions so as to adapt to the variations in the six factors of the natural environment. If these factors change abnormally or overtax the adaptability of the body, or the body's anti-pathogenic factor is weak and the vital function impaired beyond its ability to adapt itself to the changes in the weather, the occurrence of disease may depend on such factors as wind, cold, etc. which are considered pathogenic factors . . .[4]

These external pathogenic factors are obviously emphasized during the seasons, such as cold in winter. In our opinion, the cold virus can only manifest itself when the body is exposed to these external stresses and cannot adapt.

In the second century A.D., a famous Chinese physician,

Zhang Zhong Jing, wrote a medical treatise, called the *Shang-hun Lun (On Cold-Induced Disorders)*. It discusses how cold (and other factors) can penetrate and affect the body. His theory of the six stages (see Chapter Five) describes how cold penetrates in six layers, starting from the surface (*Tai Yang*) and going to the most internal levels (*Shao Yin*). The six stages is a model, not a reality, which aids the physician in deciding how to treat a patient and how seriously the illness has progressed. *Aconite* displays a picture of COLD INVASION, COLD TURNING TO HEAT, as well as disenergetic penetration to the deeper level of *shao yin* which produces fear and fright.

Belladonna: Atropha Belladonna. Solanacea.

Belladonna, also known as "deadly nightshade," is a bushy perennial that flowers in June. The flowers—single, bell-shaped blossoms with five petals—range from a reddish color to purple with a tinge of green. The plant has a dark, lurid aspect and when bruised releases a peculiar fetid odor, indicative of its narcotic nature. Every portion of the plant is poisonous. It has been responsible for the death of many a child, because the berries are shiny, black, and tantalizing. Poisoning produces a dryness of the mouth, thirst, red face, nausea, vomiting, dilated pupils, delusions, hallucinations, coma, and possible death. As a homeopathic remedy, *Belladonna* has the capacity to cure similar symptoms.

This strange plant has a long and rich history. The name, which means "beautiful woman," apparently refers to the custom of Italian women who used *Belladonna* drops to dilate their pupils for cosmetic purposes. Country folk have often associated *Bella-donna* with witchcraft, and the plant was said to be cultivated by Satan. No doubt many unsuspecting souls have fallen victim to *Belladonna*'s evil charms, and many have died because of it, but herbalists and physicians have also recognized its potential healing power, proving that virulent poisons can be converted into marvelous drugs.

Belladonna's roots and leaves have long been employed in herbal medicines from around the world. In Western herbal medicine minute doses have been used to relieve muscle pain and spasms, and it has proven to be an effective diuretic and sedative. In China, a similar species has been valued for centuries for its cooling and dispersing properties and for its efficacy in reducing pain, cooling fevers, and alleviating spasms and headaches. Modern medicine has extracted the powerful alkaloid hyoscamine from the plant; some atrophine is also present in *Belladonna*. Hyoscamine and atropine are prototypic pain killers, known in pharmacology as "antimuscarine drugs," which can block the parasympathetic nervous system.[5] Hyoscamine and atropine have immediate mild stimulating effects on the central nervous system, and a slower, longer-lasting sedative effect. In larger doses these powerful alkaloids cause excitement, delirium, headaches, facial redness, hallucinations and coma. Once again we see in these drugs a marked difference in the effect produced by the size of the doses. For instance, in tiny doses slowness of the heart beat can result, while in slightly higher doses, a fast heart beat ensues. In ancient and modern practice leaves of *Belladonna* have been used to relieve bronchial pains in asthma. Atropine and scopolamine, both solanaceceous alkaloids derived from *Belladonna*, are still used in conventional medical practice.

Keynotes and Characteristics

Homeopaths have fully explored the value of the minute dose of *Belladonna*, a major homeopathic remedy. Its value as an acute remedy is clearly defined because its symptomatology matches those of many common infectious diseases. Hahnemann had astounding success using *Belladonna* as one of his major remedies for the dreaded scarlet fever epidemics. It is commonly used for flus, earaches, sore throats and headaches if the symptoms match. Its primary symptoms include:

- A marked effect on the head and the nerves. Rapid onset of symptoms. Red and congested face, and throbbing of the affected parts. Dryness of the mouth, causing thirst. Delirium with heat and burning. Acute mania.

- Vertigo with pulsations in the head. Photophobia. Pupils dilated. Congestive headaches. Muscle spasms.
- Nausea and vomiting. Great thirst for cold water (but a dread of drinking it). Frequent and profuse urination; urine dark and turbid. Mastitis. Neck glands hot and swollen. Skin dry and hot. Boils and acne. Subjective sensation of a burning in all parts. A right-sided remedy (symptoms predominate on the right side).
- Worse: when exposed to touch, noise, or heat; in the afternoon; when sweating is checked.
- Better: when resting; when bending back.

Chinese Diagnosis

This picture of *Belladonna* is clear-cut from a Chinese point of view. The symptoms are hot, full, excessive; they potentially affect any organ or part of the body, but mostly the *liver*, *blood*, and head. *Aconite* is COLD TURNING TO HEAT; *Belladonna* is FULL HEAT. Since heat rises, many of *Belladonna*'s symptoms are in the head, such as a red face and congestive headaches. The heat can derive from outside or it can be internally generated (mostly from the LIVER IN EXCESS). *Belladonna* is a graphic picture of the internal environment succumbing to overheating.

Overcooling and overheating are two basic parameters in Chinese medicine. A person can be overheating without displaying a fever. Different diseases and people can be understood in terms of verying degrees of overheating or overcooling. Drugs and remedies can also be studied from a similar perspective. Some people tend to be vulnerable to overcooling diseases because they are constitutionally "overcooling" types with a potential to be DEFICIENT IN KIDNEY FIRE. The typical overcooling patient is thin and pale, with a soft voice, phlegmatic movements and a tendency to catch nagging colds. On the other hand, picture the typical brawny football player who eats lots of steaks (red meat—*yang*). He rarely gets sick, but when he does, it might be a fast and furious flu, perhaps accompanied by vomiting.

The Chinese doctors developed a model to explain how heat

penetrates into the body. This model of the "four stages" was discussed in Chapter Six. As heat progresses into the body, the heat signs become more pronounced and visible. For example in the third stage—*ying*—the general symptoms are: crimson to scarlet body or tongue, considerable restlessness, insomnia, a hot body, the aggravation of all symptoms at night, only slightly thirst, sometimes incoherent speech, and minute or accelerated pulses.[6] One can easily see a correlation between these symptoms and *Belladonna*.

For acute overheating conditions, the Chinese doctor might use both herbs and acupuncture to rid the heat, cool the blood, and build the *yin* (*yin* is cooling). Specific acupuncture points such as Bladder-54 (*wei yang*) and Large Intestine-11 (*wuchi*) are well known for their cooling qualities. There also are many herbs that have cooling properties. A homeopath, facing a similar situation, would have to differentiate between remedies like *Belladonna* and *Aconite*, sometimes a challenging task for the beginner.

Pyrogen

Pyrogen, or artificial sepsin, is a remedy only used in homeopathy, one of the several important *nosodes* utilized. Nosodes are remedies prepared from pathogenic or diseased tissue; if that idea seems repugnant, remember that vaccines are nosodes. Homeopathic potentization, at any rate, completely changes the nature of these substances. In the last century, homeopaths began to prove these nosodes and add them to their materia medicas. Some, like *Tuburcullinum* (from the tuberculosis nosode), are major constitutional remedies, while others, like *Pyrogen*, are used more specifically.

Pyrogen is prepared by placing a ratio of beef to water in a covered container for two weeks. This foul water is then strained and prepared into a remedy according to strict homeopathic standards. Dr. John Drysdale introduced *Pyrogen* into homeopathy in 1880. An article in the *British Medical Journal* (February 13, 1875) by Burdon Sanderson, an allopath, stimulated Drysdale's research.[7] Sanderson had used the crude *Pyrogen* to stimulate fevers in animals, and kept a careful account of the differences of fatal and near fatal doses on the animals. Without reverting to the extreme methods of his good colleague, Dr. Drysdale introduced the potentized *Pyrogen* into homeopathy.

Keynotes and Characteristics

Pyrogen is not a complex or deep remedy, but it has a clearly-delineated function and a handful of distinct keynotes—something one would expect from such an odd remedy. Its most frequent indication is acute inflammatory conditions, such as high fevers and abscesses with suppurations. In differential diagnosis *Pyrogen* must be compared with other remedies such as *Arsenicum, Anthracinum, Tarantela* and *Baptista.* Its primary indications include:

- Septic states with great restlessness and anxiety. Bursting headache. Tongue is red, dry, clean, and cracked.
- Horribly offensive discharges. Persistent vomiting. Foul diarrhea, brown or black, urgent and involuntary.
- Palpitation: pulse out of proportion to the temperature or vice-versa. Usually pulse is rapid and fever not so high. Fevers, with severe chill, begins in the small of the back. General chill of the bones and extremeties.
- Better: when becoming cold; in cold, damp weather.
- Worse: when changing positions; when exposed to heat.

Chinese Diagnosis

Pyrogen presents a fine picture of extreme internal overheating—more severe than *Belladonna. Pyrogen* is excess, *yang,* and hot; all the above keynotes indicate this. This remedy is another teaching classic, as the homeopathic indications so perfectly reflect the Chinese disharmony. One can see the myriad ways that overheating can manifest in the body: in the tongue, in the pulse, expressed in chills (extreme *yang* turning to *yin*), in the kind of headaches, or in the foul discharges. The above description of the tongue is a classic picture of overheating.

In the theory of the four stages (see *Belladonna*), Chinese

medical theory explains the invasion of external heat into the body
in four stages. In *Pyrogen* one sees the two deeper stages where
the heat begins seriously to disrupt the internal environment, producing unmistakable signs such as scarlet red tongue, restlessness,
fever, thirst, red skin eruptions and thin, rapid pulse. In some cases
of extreme overheating, the blood is damaged, producing what is
called FIRE POISON, with such symptoms as boils and carbuncles.
In the West we only associate internal overheating with high fevers
that can be registered on a thermometer, but in Chinese medicine
one sees the wide and varying range of overheating signs.

   Pyrogen and similar remedies like *Belladonna* could be said
to be the homeopathic equivalent of antibiotics. Penicillin, probably the most effective single drug devised by biochemical medicine, is a cooling drug used to combat over-heating conditions.
It follows that an overuse of penicillin and similar drugs, so common nowadays, would create an over-cooling internal environment with such symptoms as sensitivity to cold weather, susceptibility to colds and flus, and innumerable other "damp" signs. From
our knowledge of homeopathy and provings, we can see how an
abuse of penicillin might lead to a weakened resistance and in-
creased susceptibility to infection.

Veratrum Album: N.O. Melanthacea

   Veratrum, "white hellebore," is a hardy perennial with
a handsome erect stem surrounded by a cluster of greenish-white
blossoms and large curling leaves growing from the base. *Veratrum
Album*, found in Europe, has an American cousin, *Veratrum
Viride*. *Veratrum Album* is native to the mountainous regions of
Europe, and especially abundant in the Swiss Alps. The medicine
is prepared from the root.

   Veratrum Album is an ancient remedy used by Arab physicians, Dioscorides, the great Greek herbalist, and Hippocrates.
It was widely used for cerebral illness, epilepsy, mania, gout, and
eye diseases. In ancient Greece, *Veratrum* was widely used as a
purgative, to produce the evacuation and cleansing considered
essential for healing. Used carelessly, however, *Veratrum* is a

dangerous plant containing poisonous alkaloids. Hahnemann wrote an extensive paper on *Veratrum*, its history and uses, and presented this work to the faculty of the University of Leipzig. He stated that it ranked high as one of the medicines of the ancients, and also conclusively proved that the *Veratrum Album* of the ancients and the moderns is indeed the same plant.

Veratrum is not presently used in allopathic medicine because of its undependable alkaloid content and toxicity, but was still in use as recently as 1940, primarily as a cardiovascular and nerve sedative and to lower blood pressure.[8]

Characteristics and Keynotes

Veratrum Album is a unique and valuable remedy in homeopathy. The potentized drug, common in first-aid kits, produces a memorable symptom picture. *Veratrum* presents the perfect picture of collapse with extreme coldness, blueness of parts (cyanosis), and great weakness. Cold perspiration on the forehead is common. It is an excellent remedy for symptoms of post-operative shock: pale face, feeble pulse, and cold sweat on the forehead. Dr. Kent says of *Veratrum*:

> You will be astonished by the wonderful coldness running through this remedy. Hardly a group of symptoms will appear without this accompanying coldness. Coldness of discharges, coldness of the body. You would also wonder at the remarkable prostration attending the various groups of symptoms, complete relaxation, and exhaustion, coldness, profuse sweat, vomiting and diarrhea.[9]

- Other keynotes: melancholy, indifference, delirium, stupor. Delusions of impending misfortune. Mania with a desire to cut and tear things. Violent, shrieking and lewd.
- Tongue: pale and cold. Face: pale, cold, bluish.
- Voracious appetite. Thirst for cold water, immediately followed by vomiting. Rattling in the chest. Cough from cold air. Dysmenorrhea with cold sweats, vomiting and fainting.
- Worse: with least motion: at night; in cold weather; after consuming fat or beer.

- Better: in warmth; when walking; after foods; after covering
  with blankets.

Chinese Diagnosis

From the above discussion on *Veratrum*, the disharmony picture should come as no surprise. It is one of the coldest remedies
found in the homeopathic materia medica. In fact, *Veratrum*
presents a classic picture of an internal cold condition (a lack of
internal fire/*yang*). This coldness may register on the thermometer,
but more often it is detectable only from the tongue and other
symptom indicators. What is the effect on the body when the internal environment is cold? Coldness, a lack of heat and energy,
can affect virtually any function or body part. Let's briefly examine some of the symptoms that *Veratrum* produces (and therefore cures): abdominal cramps, a common symptom resulting from
cold stagnation in the middle warmer (the region of the stomach).
The vomiting results because this stagnation obstructs the normal
flow of digesting food. INTERNAL COLD STAGNATION also produces loose, watery diarrhea, the kind found in *Veratrum*. The
Veratrum patient is naturally better with warmth of any kind,
especially warm foods which heat up the stomach region.

In *Veratrum* one sees an important energetic disharmony,
called STUCK or OBSTRUCTED CHI. The harmonious flow of *chi*
in the body is a cornerstone of health. When this flow is impeded,
in this case by cold, striking symptoms of pain and discomfort
result. Everything in nature—plants, atoms, seasons, blood—is
dependent upon a continuous flow of motion; and the same is true
for *chi*. In *Veratrum* one sees the results of internal cold stagnation, and how this disharmony blocks the *chi*, food and fluids.
This obstruction is not limited to the physical plane; on the mental plane *Veratrum* manifests itself in such symptoms as stupor
and indifference. All of the symptoms produced by *Veratrum*
Album are signs of internal cold, particularly the cramps, the
vomiting, and the pain. To harmonize this COLD OBSTRUCTION
one must move the energy, dissolve the cold, and warm the body.
The Oriental doctor effects this cure with warming herbs like

ginger and capsicum, as well as acupuncture and moxabustion (a special heat therapy). From a Chinese perspective, *Veratrum Album* is a warming herb that moves cold obstruction in the middle warmer.

Dulcamera: N.O. Solanacea

Dulcamera, also known as "woody nightshade," is a wild herb common in the Eastern United States. Related to *Belladonna*, tobacco, and other nightshades, this plain shrubby plant lives in relative obscurity in damp woody areas and lacks the reputation of its more famous cousins. Sometimes mistaken for *Belladonna* because the flowers are purple, its berries are red where as those of *Belladonna* are black. Though poisonous, *Dulcamera* lacks the toxicity of *Belladonna* and its action is quite different. Active alkaloids, such as solanine, have been extracted from *Dulcamera*. Solanine is a central nervous system depressant which slows the heart beat and respiration rate, diminishes sensibility, lowers the body temperature and causes death in large doses. *Dulcamera* has no present use in conventional medicine.

In moderate doses the plant is slightly narcotic, with diuretic and diaphoretic properties. Unlike *Belladonna*, is has no effect on the eyes. In herbal medicine *Dulcamera* has an ancient history; it is mentioned by such diverse physicians as Linnaeus and the eighteenth-century Dutch physician Boerhaave. It has been used in the treatment of skin diseases, warts, ulcers, as well as chronic coughing and asthma. Presently, *Dulcamera* has little use in herbal medicine.

Keynotes and Characteristics

Dulcamera is a minor homeopathic remedy, but illustrative from the point of view of this book. Originating in the damp woods, *Dulcamera* finds its application in DAMP ailments, certain types of colds, rheumatism, and skin eruptions. The susceptible patient is often chubby, flabby, and sensitive to humid cold, and always suffers from a stuffy nose and sniffly kinds of colds.

- Back of the head is chilly or achy during cold damp weather; middle ear discharge; averse to eating, burning thirst for cold drinks.
- Mucous diarrhea, alternating green and yellow. Lumbago as if from cold, turbid urine, ill-smelling perspiration.
- Itchy and moist skin. Rheumatism worse in the muscles than the joints. Alternation between skin eruptions and intestinal or rheumatic complaints. Spongy warts.
- Better: in dry weather; when moving about.
- Worse: in cold, damp weather; at night, when resting.

Chinese Diagnosis

Like *Pyrogen*, *Dulcamera* is another gem of a remedy as it so clearly and simply depicts a Chinese disharmony pattern. We have presented the patterns of overheating and overcooling. *Dulcamera* gives us a classic picture of DAMPNESS. DAMPNESS is a very important concept in the map of internal environment, and it is not as simple as one might assume. DAMPNESS implies an excess of fluids in the tissues, such as edema, but it is a disharmony that can influence the body, any organ or part, and even the emotions and mental processes. Certain types of people are more susceptible to *damp* ailments. The stereotypic *damp* person is overweight, with a tendency to moist skin problems, weak digestion, tiredness, loose stools, and lung problems with much mucus. Just as one can go to a country where the weather is forever damp and soggy, so one can find DAMPNESS a common condition in the overall internal environment in certain individuals.

Dulcamera is primarily an acute *damp* remedy, for DAMPNESS that lodges in the body from outside; in people who tend to be chronically *damp*, however, there is often a constitutional weakness in the *spleen/stomach*, a condition we will discuss in later remedies. Almost all the signs and symptoms presented by *Dulcamera* are signs of DAMPNESS (with some heat). A *damp* skin condition will be moist, oozy, and sticky. Naturally, the *Dulcamera* person feels much better in dry, sunny weather, and worse in wet weather. During a long, damp spring with endless days of rain, the *Dulcamera* person can really suffer, and at night he will dream of a hot, dry climate like Arizona. The homeopaths were well aware of the effect of the weather and circumstances of health. Dr. Kent wrote:

> We have to observe the time of the year, the time of the day, day or night aggravations: the wet or dry remedies, the hot and cold remedies. We have to study the remedy by circumstance.[10]

On the mental/emotional plane DAMPNESS can manifest itself as lethargy, lack of spark, and mental dullness. The overall energy of the person is weighted down, more dense. One can distinctly feel the DAMPNESS in the slippery pulse, and clearly see it on the puffy tongue. DAMPNESS, acute or chronic, often mixes with other disharmonies, such as WIND and HEAT, conditions we shall see in other remedies.

Stannum

Stannum is the metal tin, an element. Tin is highly malleable and ductile but has little strength. It has been used for centuries in metal alloys for various domestic and industrial purposes, for example, to plate steel for canning food and to coat steel to preserve it from the weather. Tin is not used in conventional medicine and has rarely been used in any form of treatment. At one time it was used internally to eliminate tapeworms and externally for boils and corneal opacities.

For homeopathic use, *Stannum* must first undergo rigorous purification. Not only must it be washed thoroughly and cleaned, but heated until red hot, then washed again. This process yields a pure product, a crystalline powder. Hahnemann devised a special process, trituration, to convert metals into remedies. Instead of using a fluid for the first potencies (1x – 6x), nine grains of lactose is added to one grain of powdered tin in a mortar. This is then ground up with a pestle for one hour, producing 1x trituration of tin. One grain of this mixture is then placed in a clean mortar with nine grains of lactose and ground for one hour. After repeating this process six times (to 6x potency), it is then possible to obtain the higher potencies by the usual process of dilution and succussion. This unique process has opened the therapeutic properties of gems, minerals, and other insolubles to homeopaths.

Keynotes and Characteristics

Stannum is not a major homeopathic remedy, but one of the hundreds of minor remedies in the homeopathic materia medica. There are approximately thirty major constitutional remedies, but we will only discuss a few, like *Nux Vomica* and *Lycopodium*. For clarity, we have selected remedies with clear, simple pictures like *Stannum*. The primary picture of the *Stannum* patient is one of exhaustion of body and mind. Such an individual tires easily; he has to sit down several times while dressing in the morning, and the weakness is especially felt in the chest. Sometimes talking is a chore. Often the patient is thin and despondent; he feels like crying all the time; he is pale with respiratory weakness. Like the metal tin, a *Stannum* patient has no strength or stamina.

- Headache: begins lightly, increases gradually, then declines.
- Dizziness and weakness when descending.
- The smell of cooking causes vomiting. Sinking, "all-gone" sensation in the stomach. Colic relieved by hard pressure.
- Menses too early and too profuse. Prolapse of the uterus.
- Weak, hollow voice.
- Worse: when talking, laughing, or singing.

Chinese Diagnosis

The diagnoses in Chinese medicine are never fixed labels; they indicate a pattern that includes variables and complex interconnections. The pattern of disharmony always reflects the whole. For example, a patient with weak *lungs* (organ and meridian) might also have weakness in *kidney yang* or the *spleen*, and the practitioner is aware of these possibilities. In *Stannum* we see a simple case of DEFICIENT CHI, with a particular affinity for the *lungs*, but *chi* is always seen in relation to the *blood* and to the other major organs that effect *chi*, such as the *spleen* and *kidney*.

We chose *Stannum* because it so clearly exemplifies the disharmony pattern of DEFICIENT CHI. The *metal phase* rules the *lungs*, which bring the *chi* from the heavens into the upper warmer; there, a "sea of *chi*" forms which then blends with the *chi* generated from food to create the overall *chi* of the body. In the ancient classics the *lungs* were called the "wise judge" because they regulate the smooth and rhythmic flow of *chi* from the heavens into the body.[11] This judge offers a wide perspective of life through its knowledge of rhythm and change, and when weak the person loses perspective, withdraws, experiences grief and sadness, and is incapable of handling the changes of life.

Almost all the symptoms we see in *Stannum* relate to a weakness of *chi*, particuarly fatigue and an inability to maintain energy. The patient's voice is weak, breathing lacks stamina, and excess exertion creates difficulties. The headache of *Stannum* is a classic DEFICIENT CHI headache because it begins and ends gradually, never becoming too severe like a LIVER YANG headache. There are many factors that contribute to DEFICIENT CHI, such as improper breathing, unrelieved stress, poor diet, and overwork. DEFICIENT CHI is a common occurrence; how many times do people say, "I'm so tired this afternoon." Chronic DEFICIENT CHI is not as common. One can "read" DEFICIENT CHI in the complexion, voice, tongue, pulse, and posture.

There are other homeopathic remedies that have a strong DEFICIENT CHI picture, and some of the constitutional remedies have this disharmony within their parameters. Specific acupuncture points and herbs with tonifying properties are used to build the *chi*.

Strychonos Nux Vomica: N.O. Loganiaceae

"Poison nut," or *Nux Vomica*, is a famous, ancient medicine from the Orient. The seeds, from which the medicine is derived, grow on an evergreen tree found in China, India, and Vietnam. This tall, handsome tree produces a round fruit, as large as an orange, from which the seeds are extracted and dried. Its fame derives from the chemical content, specifically the deadly poison strychnine, one of the most potent in nature. Strychnine acts very quickly, producing violent changes in blood pressure, spasmodic respiration, convulsions, and death from asphyxia and paralysis. In moderate doses *Nux* has an interesting effect on the central nervous system, first stimulating, then depressing, finally, paralyzing.

Nux has been used for countless centuries as a medicine and a poison; it has been used, for example, to kill rodents and other pests. Like many medicines it was introduced to Europe by the Arabs in the Middle Ages, but in India and China *Nux* has a history as old as written records. Used in tiny doses, the specially-prepared seed is prescribed as a bitter stomachic (to increase the appetite), nerve tonic, laxative and spinal stimulant. *Nux*, called *ma quian zi*, is used in Chinese herbalism for its cooling, bitter, and tonic properties.[12] Presently, *Nux Vomica* has only a minor use in allopathic medicine.

Nux Vomica is a major homeopathic remedy, used for both acute and constitutional prescribing. Acute illnesses, such as the common cold, are of brief duration; constitutional illnesses are of longer duration and more complex, and therefore require more in-depth prescribing. Dr. Hahnemann discovered the inherent healing properties of this poison, rendering it harmless and incredibly curative. The whole seed is used to prepare the remedy, not just the strychnine, which is a different and less important homeopathic remedy.

Characteristics and Keynotes

Nux Vomica is a polychrest remedy, a medicine with many uses. Its symptom indicators clearly match those produced by our hectic modern life, accounting for the popularity of *Nux* in homeopathic circles. The stereotypic *Nux* patient is a quick-tempered, active male who works and plays hard. Generally, he is ambitious, practical and competitive. No doubt in this decade we will see more women needing *Nux* as they begin to fill the executive ranks. *Nux* can pursue his after-hours pleasures with equal intensity, often overindulging in food, liquor and sex. At times, he can become irritable and grouchy, with a tendency to spitefulness and cruelty. Picture the anxious boss who comes stomping into his office after a particularly late night on the town. He's impatient to get some important work done, to organize his office, but he is suffering from gastric pains, a result of the rich meal the previous night. As soon as his secretary makes a slight mistake, he snaps at her, then rushes to get a glass of water to wash down his antacid pills. Would that he would rush for the *Nux Vomica* 12x! Major keynotes include:

- Impatient; hypersensitive to spices, lights, noise and allopathic medications. Headache with vertigo, neuralgic headaches, hangovers. Takes a cold with stuffed nose. Chilly.
- Constipation with much ineffectual urging.
- Nausea, vomiting, belching, worse from rich and spicy foods.
- Craves fat and alcohol. Itching, painful hemorrhoids.
- Irregular menses with black blood. Cannot sleep after 3 a.m., and wakes up feeling wretched. Strong sexual desire.
- Better: in the evening, when exposed to warmth (except heat), after unbroken sleep, after bowel movement.
- Worse: in the early morning (around 3–4 a.m.), after eating and drinking, in cold air, after mental exertion.

Chinese Diagnosis

From a Chinese medical perspective, *Nux Vomica* also proves to be a key remedy. *Nux* presents the classic picture of CONSTRICTED LIVER CHI and LIVER YANG RISING (it is known by other names). *Nux* actually can manifest in a continuum of *liver* disharmonies, but we will keep the discussion simple here. We would like to clarify that *Nux* is not exclusively "the" medicine for liver organ diseases. LIVER YANG RISING is a disharmony picture with graphic symptoms that can affect almost any part of the body as well as the emotional and mental state. The focal point, however, of *Nux* is the *liver/gall bladder*.

In Chinese medicine the *liver* has a vastly important function that would puzzle the Western medical practitioner. The *liver*, among other functions, regulates the smooth flow of *chi* through the body/mind.[13] What happens when the *liver* cannot regulate the smooth flow of *chi*? Constriction, pain and tense muscles can result, as well as irritability, sharp local pains, headaches, wiry pulse and depression.

Another common *liver* disharmony picture arises when the LIVER FIRE or YANG becomes excessive, a common occurrence in hectic modern life. LIVER YANG RISING produces dramatic signs and symptoms: a pounding headache (often the top or side of the head), red eyes, sudden anger and shouting, loud ringing in the ears, a bitter taste in the mouth, gastric pain (*liver* commonly 'invades' the *stomach*), and a full wiry pulse (especially in the *liver* position).[14] Normally, the *liver* function is very active and is most likely to overheat, thus producing a wealth of overheating signs. The *liver* is closely related to the *gall bladder*, and in this section we will not make the fine distinctions between the two (although clinically this distinction can be crucial). The *liver* also has a close relationship with the *kidney*, particularly with the *kidney* water.

To quote from a Chinese text about the LIVER YANG disharmony picture:

> This syndrome is often due to long-standing depression of the *chi* of the LIVER which later turns to fire. Or, it may be due to indulgence in drinking and smoking causing accumulation of heat which turns to fire. The upward disturbance of the fire of the LIVER is the cause of the dizziness, distending sensation in the head, headache, red eyes, bitter taste in the mouth, and flushed face. Fire injures the *liver*, causing impairment of its function in permitting the *chi* to flow unrestrained . . .[15]

When the energy of the *liver* is harmonious, the *chi* flows smoothly through the body and there is well-being and serenity.

Another important disharmony pattern is WIND. In the internal environment, WIND signifies excess or irregular *chi*, an important clinical sign that can include itchy skin, tremors, and other involuntary movements. WIND, like DAMPNESS, OVERHEATING and OVERCOOLING, are critical energetic disharmonies in Oriental medicine, and are often hard for the Westerner initially to comprehend. Rather than analyzing them, it is best to visualize and observe them. In the case of *Nux Vomica*, WIND can result from the *liver* overheating, producing such signs as twitching muscles or wandering pains.

To someone not familiar with the energetic disharmonies of Chinese medicine, terms like LIVER YANG might seem ridiculous. Nevertheless, the universal value of these ancient Oriental observations becomes readily apparent in the clinical situation when one sees these disharmonies come to life. The Chinese long ago understood that physical ailments and emotional characteristics are closely interwoven, as in the case of LIVER YANG RISING.[16] Clearly, one can see why *Nux* is such a crucial remedy; it harmonizes the functioning of the *liver*. Modern man is inundated by stresses from all angles, with tight schedules, deadlines, traffic, finances, et. al.; concurrently, he is prone to "letting go" with alcohol, stimulants, and rich food. This lifestyle plays havoc with the *liver* and the smooth flow of *chi*, resulting in the symptoms manifest in remedies like *Nux Vomica*.

In Chinese medicine, acupuncture and herbs can be used alone or together to regulate the function of the *liver* and restore the flow of *chi*. In both systems, there are no easy formulas to treat *liver*-type conditions and people. Each case is studied individually, then treated accordingly. Certainly *Nux* is not the only remedy a homeopath would consider, as there are many remedies that affect *liver* disharmonies. Table 16 summarizes the Chinese perspective of *liver* function and disharmonies.

Lycopodium: N.O. Lycopodiacea

Often called "club moss" or "vegetable sulphur," *Lycopodium* is an evergreen moss that grows in the immense, dark, pine forests of North America and Europe. *Lycopodium*, one of many plant remedies, is unique in that it is the only representative from the moss family (one of the most ancient), a significance that might puzzle some. To those aware of the underlying phenomenon of archetypes in nature, the special potential of *Lycopodium* is

Table 16: The Liver: Different Perspectives[17]

I. The *liver* function (including meridian) according to traditional Chinese medical theory:

 1. The *liver* and meridian controls the subcostal (rib) region.
 2. It stores the *blood.*
 3. It controls the ligaments and tendons.
 4. It opens into the eyes.
 5. The meridian transverses the genital organs, lower abdomen, and subcostal region.
 6. The *liver* controls the smooth flow of *chi* throughout the body.

II. From a modern perspective we can tentatively interpret the functions and symptoms of *liver* disharmony. See the previous list for the number reference.

 1. The anatomical liver is located in the subcostal region; therefore subcostal pain is often associated with the *liver.*
 2. The liver organ receives and stores a vast amount of blood from the hepatic artery and vein. Clinical manifestation of LIVER BLOOD dysfunction include: impaired vision, loss of grasp of hands; unsteady gait; hemorrhage and menstrual disorders.
 3. The liver influences the function of the motor center. Clinical manifestations: deficiency of *liver yin* will produce wind, resulting in tremors in the hands and feet, convulsions, and numbness.
 4. In Chinese medicine the *liver* is said to effect the health of the eyes. As far as we know, there is no physiological explanation for this.
 5. The *liver* meridian is often used to treat, via acupuncture, problems along the meridian, as in the genitals.
 6. We can tentatively associate the *liver* with the functioning of the autonomic nervous system; a dysfunction in either has a profound effect on the emotional state. *Liver* dysfunction produces irritability, anger, distention in the chest and muscular tension, such as a sensation of a lump in the throat.

apparent. A major homeopathic remedy, *Lycopodium* evokes a unique constellation of physical and mental characteristics that finds a powerful resonance in the world of men and women.

In herbalism *Lycopodium* has found intermittent use through the course of history, but nowadays it is rarely found outside of homeopathic circles. The full curative potential of the plant is only released by potentization. In Europe, however, the plant has found sporadic use as a diuretic and liver remedy. The Druids reputedly used a similar species as a powerful cathartic for purging the bowels.[18] In Germany dry *Lycopodium* spores were used to create false lightning in theaters, hence the name "vegetable sulphur." In pharmacies the powder was used as a drying agent to coat pills. The yellowish spores, from which the remedy is prepared, float on water and are suprisingly flammable. Generally considered medically inert, the discovery of *Lycopodium* is another testimony to the genius of Samuel Hahnemann—as any practicing homeopath will readily concur. Hahnemann, for some unknown reason (there were obviously hundreds of potential remedies to test), decided to prove Lycopodium and discovered a medicinal gold mine. Presently, *Lycopodium* is a major remedy for constitutional and acute prescribing.

Keynotes and Characteristics

In provings *Lycopodium* yielded a wide range of symptoms, affecting all organ systems and displaying a graphic picture. The stereotypic *Lycopodium* is thin, with a sallow, lined face, keen intellect, weak muscular power, and a host of digestive problems like swelling of abdomen after eating and flatulence. Though professionally capable, the adult *Lycopodium* often presents a bold exterior hiding a nagging self-doubt. He is prone to lack of confidence, insecurity, irritability, fear of new situations and fear of failure. George Vithoulkas, the reknowned Greek homeopath, describes the emotional core of *Lycopodium* as pervasive cowardice; it requires the astute homeopath to spot the *Lycopodium* because of his bombastic facade. In the homeopathic repertory one finds *Lycopodium* as the only remedy listed under the heading, "the love of power." Because of their deep lack of confidence, *Lycopodium* patients love to be in a position of power, and because they are often intellectual, they can be found in successful professional positions. For example: An important politician, at the height of his career, falls into a sudden crisis of confidence after a period of prolonged work. Suddenly, he finds that he is terrified at the prospect of facing a political rally. *Lycopodium* is one major remedy to consider in cases of fear of facing a crowd. This remedy demonstrates a strong psychological component and a distinct counterpart of physical symptoms. The chronic *Lycopodium* patient, left untreated, can eventually suffer from memory loss, impotence, bad temper, and chronic depression.

- A right-sided remedy, with symptoms often worse between four and eight p.m.
- Irritable; malicious; wants to be alone, yet dreads solitude.
- Headaches come on with gastric problems; furrowed brow; premature balding; constipation, flatulence, and sour eructations. Sour taste in the mouth. Pain in the liver region.
- Craves sweets.
- Premature ejaculation; frequent urination at night.
- Psoriasis. One foot remains hot, the other, cold (a good example of a useful peculiar symptom).
- Feels better from warm food and drinks.

Chinese Diagnosis

Like all constitutional remedies, *Lycopodium* is difficult to categorize, but there is a definite pattern of disharmony discernible in this remedy. In general *Lycopodium* is *yin*, cold, and deficient. There is a lack of *chi* and *blood*, and a particular affinity for the *liver* and *kidney* (also, *stomach* and *intestine*.) The center of gravity in this remedy is the *liver* and *gall bladder*. *Lycopodium* makes an interesting contrast to *Nux Vomica* which is more confident, aggressive, and robust. *Nux* is an excess *liver* remedy, *Lycopodium* is a deficient *liver/gall bladder* remedy. The irritability, sourness, and digestive problems stem from this WOOD DISHARMONY INVADING STOMACH AND INTESTINES. There are signs of LIVER

BLOOD DEFICIENCY in the dry skin and depression with cranki-
ness.[19] In China it is often said that a person with courage has
a big, healthy gall bladder; one could say the opposite of *Lycopodium*.

The full spectrum of *Lycopodium* cannot be fully understood
without studying the meridians intimately connected to the *wood*
phase, with special emphasis here on the *kidneys*. KIDNEY YIN
nourishes the *liver*. In fact, in advanced *Lycopodium* cases one sees
a deficiency of both KIDNEY YIN and YANG. When the KIDNEY
YANG is weak, one finds a lack of vital fire, resulting in such symptoms as impotence, premature ejaculation, pervasive insecurity
and fears, and a sensitivity to cold—all classic *Lycopodium* symptoms. The *kidney* energy is said to be the foundation of *yin* and
yang, the very core of the drive and strength of the body and mind.
In the chronic stages of *Lycopodium* disharmony, one sees a sad
picture of a deep *liver/kidney* deficiency: fearful, cranky person;
impotent, dry-skinned and prematurely old; he wants isolation
yet also fears it.

Lachesis

Lachesis is a remedy prepared from the venom of a
deadly snake, the "bushmaster" (*surucucu*), found only in the
Amazon jungle. The venom has a paralyzing effect on the nerves,
directly weakens the brain and heart, decomposes the blood (like
most snake poisons) and inevitably causes death. Nearly all provings were made in potencies 30c or higher. Two other snake venoms—rattlesnake and cobra—are converted into homeopathic
remedies, but *Lachesis* is the most important.

Lachesis is an intriguing remedy because of its exotic origin,
curious history, marked healing power and symbolic/psychological
significance. Unknown to any medical system but homeopathy,
Lachesis was discovered by the great homeopathic scientist and
doctor, Constantine Hering. Dr. Hering, a student of Hahnemann,
moved from Germany to America in the middle of the last century
and became a leader in homeopathy in America. In 1828, while
still in Germany, he was sent by the German government to study

the flora and fauna of the Amazon basin.[20] Hering, famous for his scientific ardor, became determined to capture the notorious bushmaster. As the story goes, he offered a reward to the local people to bring forth the dreaded snake. After some delay, a snake was reluctantly delivered in a bamboo box. Everyone, including the servants, fled the jungle camp, leaving Hering and his wife with the snake. Unperturbed, he stunned the snake with a blow from a club and cautiously extracted venom, but the effect of just preparing the remedy threw him into delirium and mania—the venom being so potent—much to the dismay of his wife who then nursed him through the night. Waking from a coma the next morning, he was interested only in the effect of the remedy on his body and mind. Reputedly, he opened his eyes and asked his wife to record what he had done and said (so keen was he to learn symptoms of this potential remedy).

Later, *Lachesis* was proved in a more official manner and added to the homeopathic materia medica where it was established as a major constitutional remedy. In all medical systems, virulent poison can be converted into potent medicines. But only in homeopathy, with its unique method of dilution and succussion, can poisons be rendered so safe and curative.

Keynotes and Characteristics

Lachesis is a deep and complex remedy producing, and therefore curing, a wide range of symptoms. Dr. Kent, the American homeopath, prefaces his discussion of *Lachesis* with the following words:

> *Lachesis* seems to fit the whole human race, for the race is pretty filled up with the snake as to disposition and character and this venom only causes to appear what is in man.[21]

The snake has been a powerful symbol through all history and finds striking representation in every major culture. It is a symbol of the primordial and impersonal life energy, of the libido, and of the drive for sex and survival. The price man inevitably pays for his personal development is the isolation and repression of vital forces such as the libido.[22] In psychology the libido is seen as the unconscious drive for life, pleasure and sex, and in *Lachesis* there is a suppression of and conflict with the libido. This potent instinct, indeed the root of life, must be sacrificed for the needs and pressures of self and society. *Lachesis* is an archetype, or model, of this universal conflict: man's struggle with the libido.

The general picture of the *Lachesis* type is dramatic and turbulent, somewhat like a character out of a nineteenth-century Russian novel.[23] The *Lachesis* type can have all or some of the following characteristics: He may be brilliant, intuitive, loquacious, sharp tongued, swayed by suspicion and hatred, envious, and in extreme cases ruled by cruel impulses and delusions. For instance, religious insanity can occur; a woman, for example, may believe that she is under superhuman control. The individual can experience flights of imagination, ecstatic states, or hallucinations. The *Lachesis* may be manic depressive, going from one extreme to another, from fits of gambling and drinking to fits of self-humiliation and denial. Of course, sexuality can be a strong driving force, sometimes excessive, sometimes suppressed. *Lachesis* individuals can be depraved drunks, religious zealots, brilliant writers, and great politicians. On a less extreme level the *Lachesis* type is sensual, lively, humorous and a great talker, but always battling the dualistic struggle within. Other keynotes include:

- Hot flashes; hot pressure and burning on the top of the head; hammering of headaches as if the head would burst; migraines.
- Great sensitivity to touch; clothes cause discomfort on the skin. Intolerant of tight bands around the neck.
- Sense of constriction in various parts. All of these symptoms are worse after sleep. Wounds bleed easily.
- Tonsilitis or sore throat: begins on the left side, extends to the right; the throat has a dark purple appearance. Tongue swollen and trembling. Cold hands and feet result from the slightest exertion.
- Affinity for the ovaries in the female, especially the left side. Menopause. The menses are always better when the flow

commences. Generally, *Lachesis* improves with discharges.
- Better: in the open air, after cold drinks.
- Worse: in the morning; when awakening, after alcohol, when exposed to extreme temperatures.

Chinese Diagnosis

What immediately stands out in *Lachesis* is constriction, heat, and "troubled spirit." The *Lachesis* patient presents an interesting duality of *liver* and *heart* disharmonies. The constriction of *liver* stands out, manifesting in physical tensions and a multitude of muscular constrictons. There is an interplay of *liver* constriction, *liver* and *heart* overheating, and *shen* problems. *Shen* (loosely defined as "personality") problems indicate emotional and mental struggles and conflicts. The *Lachesis* patient is very different from the stolid, phlegmatic *Calcarea*, and is more volatile than the irritable *Nux vomica*.

In *Lachesis*, the *chi, blood*, and *liver* energy are bottled up. Sporadically this containment surges out in some physical, emotional or mental outlet such as loquaciousness, anger, bursting headaches, hot flashes, or excess bleeding. The *liver*, as we have explained, controls the smooth flow of *chi* in the *body/mind* and it stores the *blood;* both of these functions can therefore be perverted in *Lachesis*. The musculature can be tense and any constriction of clothing can be annoying, both signs of *liver* constriction. From a modern Chinese text one sees the following signs of LIVER CONSTRICTION and LIVER YANG EXCESS.

> Distension and pain in the subcostal regions, oppression and discomfort in the chest, irritability, dysmenorrhea, sensation of pharygeal obstruction, pain and distention in the breast and lower abdomen, flushed face, congested eyes, bowstring pulse, and quick temper.[24]

Lachesis patients manifest these symptoms right down to the detail of the sensation of constriction in the throat, a classic *Lachesis* symptom. In Chinese medicine, the *heart* governs the *blood* and in rest the *liver* stores the *blood,* two functions which are perverted in *Lachesis.* Constriction of the *chi* can affect the *blood* and the menses, causing discomfort and pain. As a result, *Lachesis* generally improves with any discharges. the *Lachesis* woman, for example, is better after menstrual flow because the tension of containment is released. This principle is also true on the emotional and mental levels. For instance, *Lachesis* is a major remedy for people who talk excessively.

As we explain in regard to the next remedy, *Aurum,* the *heart* stores the *shen.* In *Lachesis* there are *shen* problems, including a wide variety of emotional problems such as jealousy and hatred. In Chinese medicine any impairment of the *heart* spirit will result in insomnia, amnesia, psychosis, hallucination and other disorders of consciousness.[25] Interestingly, the *liver* and *heart* have an intimate five-phase connection in Chinese medicine. The *liver* is the "mother" of the heart because it nourishes the heart. One might say that in *Lachesis* these is a conflict between the *liver* and the *heart* because the *liver* is said to store the "animal spirit" (instinct) and the heart stores the "spirit" (personality), and as we have inferred, *Lachesis* represents the conflict between instinct and personality.

Aurum Metallicum

Aurum is a metallic gold. It needs little introduction, for gold has seduced and fascinated man since it was first extracted from the earth. It is well loved for its beauty and for its monetary value. As one might expect, gold is an intriguing homeopathic remedy, one of many metallic remedies used in homeopathy. Gold is one of the few metals occurring in nature in its pure form. It is an extremely unreactive metal, insoluble in water, nitric, and sulphuric acids.

In medical history, gold has a long but inconsistent history. Many traditional medicines, such as Ayurvedic practice in India, employed the potential healing power of gold. In Ayurvedic medicine gold is used as a gem elixir, for reasons we will grasp after reading this section. The great Arabian physicians of the middle

ages, at the height of the Arab renaissance, understood the healing power of gold. In the beginning of the eleventh century,
Avicenna (canon, Lib. II, Cap. 79) said:

> Powdered gold is added to medicines against melancholy;
> it cures fetid odor of the mouth, and taken internally, it is even
> curative of falling out of hair; it strengthens the eyes, helps car-
> dialgia and palpitation of the heart, and is extremely useful in
> asthma.[26]

Hahnemann seemed to take his cue from the Arabs, ignoring the
skepticism of his contemporaries, and experimented with gold as
a remedy, the secret being the preparation of diluted potency so
there are no toxic side effects. Hahnemann says:

> I believe that I might well prefer the testimony of the Ara-
> bians concerning the curative virtues of fine powder of gold to
> the theoretical doubts of the moderns supported by no experi-
> ment: I therefore rubbed the finest leaf-gold (of 23 carat, 6 grain
> fineness) with 100 parts of sugar of milk for a full hour, in order
> to apply it to internal medicinal use.[27]

With homeopathic provings the work of the Arabs was verified
and expanded, and gold became a great homeopathic remedy,
especially valuable for states of suicidal depression.

In its pure state gold is considered medicinally inert. Homeopathy predates the modern medical use of gold salts. In current
allopathic medicine gold salts, such as gold sodium thiomalate,
are used for rheumatoid arthritis; the mechanism of its physiological action is a mystery. Gold thus used is excreted by the kidneys.
All gold compounds are potentially toxic, capable of producing
dizziness, fainting, sweating, flushing, malaise, nausea, and weakness; less common are syncope, bradycardia, thickening of the
tongue, difficulty breathing and swallowing as well as various skin
reactions, all crude provings of gold. Besides being non-toxic, the
homeopathic gold has a much broader and deeper action.

In alchemy gold represents the *yang* life force, the blood, the
warmth, the vitality, and the life in the heart. This precious metal

owes its underlying attraction to this symbolic force. Gold is the sun of metals. In metals gold is the great representation of life force. The *yin* aspect of gold, the "black sun," is the degenerative form that symbolizes the antithesis of the solar principle as it signifies decay, lack of life and emotion (the *Aurum* picture).[28]

Characteristics and Keynotes

Dr. Burnett, the British homeopath, went to the extent of proving homeopathic *Aurum* on himself, reasoning that, "to get a concrete conception of what a drug can do, there is nothing like trying it on your own body."[29] On the first day after it had taken effect, he experienced exhilaration, but in a few days depression and low spirits set in. "Nothing seems worthwhile," Burnett wrote. He experienced nightmares, dreaming of death, of the dead, and of corpses. And "fearing the effects in this direction might be serious," [30] he quickly antidoted the proving, concluding, "I am thoroughly satisfied that [gold] can make me ill. My allopathic brethren maintain that gold is inert! Sure proof that they have never tried it, properly triturated, on their own bodies."[31]

Gold has a profound effect on mental and emotional states, producing depression, suicidal impulses, apathy, utter self-condemnation, and a disgust for life. There can be a hurriedness in the actions, irritability, and oversensitivity to noise. In the body gold can have a devastating effect, attacking the blood, the glands, and the bones, conditions that can bear a strong resemblance to syphilitic (and mercurial) infections. Other symptoms include:

- Dejection; longings for death; the thought of death gives great joy.
- Violent pain in the head; worse at night. Extreme photophobia; pressure and tension in the eyes. The patient sees double. Upper half of objects invisible.
- Heart palpitations, angina, sensation as if the heart had stopped beating for a few seconds. Feeble and irregular pulse.
- Back pains and deformities; arthritic conditions.

Chinese Diagnosis

The bioenergetic essence of gold as a therapeutic agent is fascinating, and like the precious metal, medicinal gold is a powerful substance. Looking at the symptoms revealed by homeopathy, gold is clearly a *heart* remedy. Gold treats the heart organ, but more importantly it treats the emotions related to the *heart*. The *Su Wen* states, "The *heart* rules *blood* and blood vessels," and "the *heart* stores the *shen*."[32] These are the two primary functions of the *heart* according to Oriental medical theory. *Shen*, an elusive concept to convey in the English language, is best translated as the "spirit," or even more loosely, the "personality." *Shen* is the spirit that makes each one of us a unique, thinking and feeling person.[33] In the West we more readily say that *shen* is the brain, a pure intellectual function, but in most traditional medicines the *heart* is recognized as the "house" of our emotional/mental function. When the *shen* is not nourished, one sees symptoms like poor memory, forgetfulness, insomnia, restlessness, and in extreme cases hysteria, madness, and incoherent speech.[34]

In Chinese medicine it is well understood that the mind and body are interconnected. *Aurum*, with its severe *shen* disturbance, indicates a disruption in this connection. The love of life and affection has been sadly eroded. *Heart* and *shen* problems are intimately connected. In Chinese medicine the *heart* is associated with the emotion of joy, a quality lacking in the *Aurum* person. One also sees heart organ problems such as palpitations, listlessness, and irregular pulse. Other physical manifestations include bone problems and arthritis (the allopathic use)—a physical manifestation (degeneration) of mental/emotional erosion.

The center of gravity of *Aurum* is the *heart* and the *shen*, but one also sees serious problems affecting other organ systems, especially the *kidney* and *liver*. Eye problems are common (*liver* governs the eyes); the eyes are said to be "the window of the *shen*." The *Aurum* person is lacking in vital heat (*yang*) which manifests in the *kidney* and *heart yang;* they are blood deficient, and cold both emotionally and physically.

Calcarea Carbonia: CALCIUM CARBONATE

Calcarea Carbonia, one of the great homeopathic remedies, is prepared from the inner shell of the oyster, a seemingly inert substance. John Henry Clark, M.D., the famous British homeopath, wrote about *Calcarea:*

> "*Calcarea* is one of the greatest monuments of Hahnemann's genius. His method of preparing insoluble substances brought to light in this instance a whole world of therapeutic power formerly unknown. Moreover, *Calcarea* is one of the polychrest remedies, and ranks with *Sulphur* and *Lycopodium*. . . . All three have a very wide range and deep action."[35]

"Polychrest" signifies remedies of broad and deep action. Calcium is an extremely important mineral on this earth and in our bodies. It is the fifth most abundant element in the human body, preceded ony by hydrogen, oxygen, nitrogen and carbon. It is a major component of the bones and teeth, plays a role in the cellular permeability to potassium and sodium ions, and is also responsible for the contraction and retraction of the muscles.

It is interesting to note that oyster shell is an important remedy in Chinese medicine, used for calming the spirit and building the *yin*. It is used for such symptoms as night sweats, irritability, dizziness and insomnia.

Because the enormous therapeutic value of *Calcarea* is best released through potentization, conventional medicine recognizes its use only in the minor role as an antacid and mineral supplement. There is an immense gap between the allopathic and homeopathic use of this substance. Homeopathy uses *Calcarea* as a major constitutional remedy, stimulating the body to function properly on all levels.

Keynotes and Characteristics

Improper assimilation of food is one of the keynotes of homeopathic *Calcarea,* and one of the major causes of disease predisposition. The *Calcarea* patient is often pale, plump, and flabby, unable to assimilate calcium (and other nutrients) from his food, and can have problems with bone formation—more common in early childhood. Potentized *Calcarea* can correct this condition. *Calcarea* is an excellent remedy for children who are fat, prone to chills, and suffering from slow bone formation. Emotionally, the *Calcarea* type of person is slow, cautious, stubborn, prone to feel vulnerable to the world, and like the oyster tends to project a wall around himself. He tires easily, sweats profusely (especially on the head at night), eats a lot and goes through life methodically. Other major indications include the following:

- Forgetful; many fears; slow; dependable; broods over little things; indolent; slow of mind.
- Vertigo, especially in high places. Obesity. Large head and abdomen. Curvature of the spine. Lacks vital heat. Catches a cold at every change of weather.
- Craves indigestible things: chalk, pencils, dirt. Craves sweets, eggs; dislikes fats. Sour eructation; sour sweat. Aversion to milk.
- Menses too early and too profuse. Sexual lassitude.
- Constipation, then diarrhea. Rheumatic condition of the joints. Sleepless with cold extremities. Tendency to warts. In children problems with teething, anemia, rickets, tuberculosis.
- Worse: with exertion; when ascending; when exposed to cold, water, moist air, wet weather, or the full moon; when standing.
- Better: in dry climate and weather; when lying on the painful side, sneezing.

Chinese Diagnosis

Calcarea presents a very different picture from the *liver*-type remedies we have just discussed. *Calcarea* is an "earth" type of remedy, focusing on the *spleen/stomach*, the energy centers that process food into energy (therefore involving several anatomical organs). When this transformative function is impaired, food is not properly digested and assimilated, the energy becomes deficient, and the production of "low grade material" results: phlegm, mucus, fat, diarrhea.[36] Other symptoms include lethargy, digestive weakness, tendency to gain weight, fluid problems, mental and physical torpor and perspiration—all signs of "dampness," and all keynotes of *Calcarea*. Like *Dulcamera, Calcarea* is a DAMP remedy but on a more profound level. Both these remedies feel better in dry weather.

An important concept in Chinese medicine is the *triple warmer*, the meridian and function that governs the metabolism of water and food in what we call the "three warmers." The three warmers (or "heaters") are three energetic sections of the torso. The first is basically the thoracic cavity, lungs and heart. Below the diaphragm is the middle warmer, spleen, stomach and liver—the digestive segment. The lower warmer consists of the intestines, kidney, bladder and genital organs. The coordination of these three warmers is governed by the *triple warmer* function. In *Calcarea* one sees a weakness in the middle warmer which can affect the other warmers or any part of the body.

In Chinese medicine the three functions most responsible for the production of *chi* are the *lungs, spleen,* and *kidney yang*. These functions are reflected in the right hand pulses and together are called the *chi* pulses (the left hand pulses are called the *blood* pulses). If the *spleen chi* is weak one might expect to see a weakness in the *lungs* and *kidneys*. For instance, in a *lung* condition with much coughing and mucus, the underlying weakness can be in the *spleen*, because it is the generator of excess mucus. To treat only the *lungs* would be temporary palliation. The *lungs* introduce the *chi* from the air into the body, the *spleen* and *stomach* produce *chi* from food. The *kidney fire* is said to be the "pilot light" of the earth (*spleen*/stomach). The *kidney* symptoms are bone problems, lower back pain, edema, sexual disfunctions, fears and chilliness.[37] *Calcarea* patients are notoriously susceptible to cold, drafts, and dampness. They tend to be slow, phlegmatic people; they do things step by step and are not impulsive and quick like the *Nux Vomica* people. The *damp* quality affects the state of mind, producing such symptoms as lethargy, a tendency to mull over details, stubbornness, inability to concentrate, and inflexibility.

In *Calcarea* one sees a DEFICIENCY OF FIRE and an EXCESS OF DAMPNESS, resulting from SPLEEN and KIDNEY FIRE DEFICIENCY. From a Western physiological aspect, one could relate this *fire* quality to the adrenals, which secrete the activating hormones of "fight and flight"; to the thyroid, which governs metabolism; and to sex hormones.

Let's briefly look at a *Calcarea* patient. A twenty-three year old female comes to our clinic complaining of partial deafness, excess weight, and fluid retention. She's a single mother, timid and quiet, with a tendency to over-sympathize (a *spleen* type of emotion); she lacks confidence and still lives with her parents. Her body is slightly overweight; she has a pale tongue and complexion, and she tends to complain. Her medical doctor has told her that she has a tendency to build up fluid in the middle ear which is the cause of her partial deafness. Her pulses are slippery and slow. She gets colds easily and her abdomen tends to bloat during her menstrual period. She has a pretty face, fair complexion and a gentle manner. After a full diagnosis we see that she is deficient in her *spleen* and *kidney* energy. She is a *damp* kind of person, and a candidate for *Calcarea*. From a Chinese medical perspective the essence of *Calcarea* is a lack of transformative fire.

One of the many enigmas that confronts Westerners when they first study Chinese medicine is the correlation between energy functions and seemingly unrelated tissue. For example, the *kidneys* are said to govern the bones; the *spleen*, the flesh; the *liver*, the tendons. Bone problems can often be related to a *kidney* dysfunction. Likewise, problems with the muscles and flesh are often related to the *earth phase (spleen/stomach)*. For instance, an excess of flesh can result from an incomplete transformation of food into energy. It's logical to assume that the function which governs the transformation of food into energy and flesh also "governs" the flesh. The relationship of *Calcarea* to metabolism and the muscles is also an interesting one. The mineral calcium (*Calcarea*) is crucial to the proper functioning of the muscles. If the absorption of nutrients, particularly calcium, is inhibited for any reason, the muscles will not be nourished, producing flabby, atonic muscles—a *damp* symptom or *Calcarea* keynote.

Mercurius Vivus: **Mercury**

Mercury, a well-known metal, has a unique quality—at room temperature it is a liquid. Mostly found in chemical compounds, mercury is extremely toxic, making it a major environmental hazard. Its homeopathic potentization, however, yields a powerful healing medicine. The use of crude mercury, one of the major drugs of the last century, has a long and infamous history in allopathic medicine. When George Washington was sick with the flu, his physicians not only bled him excessively but also administered immoderate doses of calomel, a mercury compound. He never made it through the night! For many decades mercury masqueraded as a wonder drug, and it did seem to be useful in the treatment of syphilis for which conventional medicine had no other alternatives. Today, practitioners of allopathic medicine, realizing its potential toxicity, only use mercury in topical compounds such as mercurachrome and fungacides. Even its use in dental fillings is beginning to be questioned.

Mercury poisoning leads to symptoms similar to those seen in syphilis. Consequently, this property led to its use in the homeopathic treatment of syphilis, when the totality of symptoms match. Dr. Hahnemann, also a chemist, produced a unique form of mercury, black oxide, which became the dominant form used in allopathic preparations even to this day.

Characteristics and Keynotes

Mercurius is a popular homeopathic remedy, used in both constitutional and acute prescribing. The constitutional *Mercurius* type is flabby, fat, sweaty, and foul smelling, with fetid discharges and breath—not a pretty picture! Just as mercury, the metal, is used in thermometers to measure temperature, the *Mercurius* patient is similarly sensitive to hot and cold. There is a lack of vitality and warmth, yet the patient suffers from the heat of his bed at night. There is much trembling, suppuration, ulceration, and commonly the patient splutters and salivates while speaking. He will catch a cold easily and is sensitive to drafts and humidity. *Mercurius* is the best representative of Hahnemann's "syphlitic miasm," one of his three primary classifications of disease.

The *Mercurius* personality is dualistic. On one hand there is the *yin* type: morose, anxious, guilty, timid, and disgusted with life. On the other hand, we have the *yang* type, a rogue, a gangster, violent, cruel, impulsive, and "pushed to destroy those he loves best." In the middle we find a hasty, nervous person who has trouble finding a place in society. These people often have weak memories, make simple arithmetical errors, and are prone to fetid discharges. Susceptible children are those who go around touching everything, talking very fast, and with a tendency to stammer. Other keynotes include:

- Impulsive, mistrustful, feeble-willed.
- Thick yellow discharges from the ears. Dirty-looking faces. Glands inflamed and swollen.
- Tooth decay; black teeth. Tongue large and flabby with yellow coat and indentation of teeth. Swollen bleeding gums. Soreness; burning; swelling in the throat; burning in throat, as from hot vapor ascending.
- Painful ulcers. Dysentary: stools slimy, bloody, and foul. Loss of appetite with a metallic taste. Intense thirst with profuse perspiration. Disordered digestion. Aversion to sweets, beer, greasy foods, butter, milk.
- Pale, clotted, acrid menstral flow. Acrid burning vaginal discharges. Excess urination, often burning.
- Fever with creeping chilliness. Sweats day and night without relief.
- Moist oozing eruptions. Inflammations and rheumatism. Tendency to form boils. Trembling of extremities, especially the hands.
- Worse: at night; in damp weather; when lying on the right side, perspiring, or in a warm room or bed.
- Better: with bed rest; when exposed to moderate temperatures.

Chinese Diagnosis

Dulcamera and *Calcarea* manifest many typical *damp* signs with minor displays of heat. In *Mercurius* we see the classic DAMP HEAT remedy. We have already discussed the disharmonies of overheating and of dampness in some detail; together, overheating and dampness produce DAMP HEAT, of which there are differing degrees of severity. Dampness is *yin*, watery, and slow; heat is hot, active, and *yang*. DAMP HEAT is reminiscent of being stuck in Boston traffic on a hot humid August day. The combination of damp and heat in the body produces the rather disagreeable symptoms we see in *Mercurius*. *Mercurius* is noted for foul discharges, a key sign of serious DAMP HEAT conditions. As we discussed in the case of *Dulcamera*, dampness can invade from the outside and lodge in the tissue, but in *Mercurius* it is more commonly the result of an internal disharmony producing a DAMP HEAT condition. Internal DAMP HEAT can result from several factors such as diet, excess alcohol and disharmonies of the *spleen*, *kidney* and *liver*. Because of its adverse effect on the *spleen* and *liver*, alcohol produces DAMP HEAT. DAMP HEAT can affect any part of the body and can be involved in numerous disease categories. For instance, some kinds of arthritis display distinct DAMP HEAT characteristics such as hot, fluid-filled, painful joints. The DAMP HEAT symptoms of *Mercurius* are lingering, heavy, oozing, fetid, thick, and yellow ("yellow" signifies heat, while "clear" or "white" signifies cold). Skin ulcerations with oozing, yellowish discharges are a sign of DAMP HEAT that is discharging through the skin. In a typical DAMP HEAT condition, as we see in *Mercurius*, one can expect to find a weak *spleen* producing the dampness, as well as an overheating *liver*. An overheating damp condition can also exist in the *intestines*, the *kidneys*, and the *bladder*. Generally, the DAMP HEAT condition presented by *Mercurius* is a chronic condition, but *Mercurius* also has important use in acute conditions such as the oozing yellow ear discharge common in children.

The homeopathic texts provide a vivid picture of the *Mercurius* tongue: It is large, flabby, coated with yellow and indented.

This detailed description of the tongue is surpassed in medical literature only by the Chinese. The *Mercurius* tongue is identical to the DAMP HEAT tongue described in Chinese medicine.[38] The *Mercurius* tongue graphically demonstrates the changes DAMP HEAT will produce on the tongue, its shape, coating and color.

Selenium: The Element Selenium

Selenium is a rare, non-metallic element, closely related to sulphur and found in many chemical combinations with it. *Selenium* was discovered in 1817 by the famous chemist, John Berylius, while he was studying a method of producing sulphuric acid. It is a lustrous reddish-brown substance, amorphous, brittle and non-soluble in water or alcohol. Like sulphur, it burns, but the odor of *Selenium* is more like horseradish.

Selenium has never been used in Chinese or Western herbalism, and it has no use in biochemical medicine except as an ingredient in fungicides and recently as a mineral supplement. It was the first semiconductor discovered; therefore, it is crucial to the electronics industry. Because its resistance is directly affected by light, it is an important element in photoelectric cells. In the gaseous form *Selenium* is quite toxic, and concentrations above ten parts per million are considered deadly. This is an example of the minute dose having a physiological effect. (Conventional medicine has always scorned homeopathy for its use of the minute dose.) *Selenium* is particularly toxic to the *liver, lungs* and *kidneys*. Nonetheless, it is an essential trace element in the body, especially in the bones, teeth and the testicles.[39] It works synergistically with Vitamin E since they are both antioxidants, preventing or at least slowing down the hardening of tissue and aging. Males appear to need *Selenium* more than women, since it is lost through ejaculation of the semen. *Selenium* works with Vitamin E in some of its metabolic actions, promoting normal body growth and fertility.

Keynotes and Characteristics

Selenium was first proved by Dr. Constantine Hering in the last century. Once again the homeopaths antedated modern biochemical knowledge in their use of *Selenium*. It is not a major remedy, but it has a distinct picture, useful when well-indicated. The *Selenium* patient is frequently light-complexioned, forgetful, easily exhausted and prone to impotence. He always wants to sleep but sleep does not refresh him. His skin may be greasy and shiny, with numerous blackheads, and the hair on his head falls out easily. These symptoms are more common in older people.

- Weak memory; easily fatigued. Extreme sadness. Lascivious thoughts with impotence; hunger at nighttime. Hoarseness of singers. Premature ejaculations. Dribbling of semen or urine. Weak or ill-humored after coitus.
- Worse: with alcohol or coffee; when exposed to drafts, exertion, sun, heat.
- Better: after inhaling cool air, taking rest; after sunset.

Chinese Diagnosis

Selenium, a marvelous picture of a DEFICIENT KIDNEY function, must be understood in some detail because it is so vital to the energetic map of the body. In Western medicine the kidneys are seen as two relatively small organs in the lower back that filter and control the fluid balance in the body. The Chinese concept of the *kidneys* includes this definition and more. The *kidneys* are said to be the foundation of the *yin* and *yang* in the body. There are two aspects to the *kidneys, kidney yin* and *kidney yang*. The *kidney yin* partially relates to the water and cleansing function of the *kidneys;* the *kidney yang* is related to their active or firey aspect.

The *kidney yang* is said to be the source of the "fire" of the body, so crucial for metabolism, warmth, and countless other activities. Sexual vigor is related to the *kidney yang*. The *kidney yang* can be related to several endocrinal secretions such as adrenaline, related to the fight-or-flight response, the sexual hormones, and the thyroid hormones, which regulate metabolism. *Kidney yang* also corresponds with the Hindu concept of the lower *chakras*, or energy centers, relating to sex and survival. In the five-phase correspondences, we see that the *kidneys* are related to the bones;

the teeth; the hearing; the salty flavor; mental concentration; the emotion of fear; wintertime; urine, and the bladder; and the hair on the head. When the *kidney yang* is in serious disharmony, an individual may develop uncontrollable fears (phobias), weak bones, intense dislike of cold weather (lack of fire), as well as urinary problems. In *Selenium* we see a graphic picture of depletion of the *kidney chi* (not the *kidney yang*). The great majority of symptoms expressed by *Selenium* in homeopathic texts are symptoms of DEFICIENT KIDNEY CHI.

Studying a remedy like *Selenium* in the context of Chinese and homeopathic traditions clearly supports the major thesis of this book: In the bioenergetic concept of illness, discernible patterns of disharmony emerge that are described by different names in these two distinct systems. Even more incredibly, we see remarkably correlations not only between the homeopathic *Selenium* and KIDNEY CHI weakness, but with the modern biochemical knowledge of the trace element *Selenium* as well. We must reiterate that the homeopathic knowledge of *Selenium* predates this century, long before the crucial functions of the element *Selenium* were clearly understood. Over one hundred years ago homeopathic doctors started to use *Selenium* to alleviate symptoms of impotence, fatigue, aging and weak memory.[40] Only in the past thirty years, however, has biochemical research begun to reveal that this trace element is a key antioxidant in the body and has a crucial role in maintaining health; a deficiency of *Selenium* is implicated in impotence, premature aging, and higher rates of cancer. In fact, the element is found in the hair, testicles, bones and teeth—all related to the *kidney* energy![41] Chinese doctors, with their careful observation of sick and healthy people, would well understand the symptoms presented by *Selenium*. The *Selenium* patient is weak; he fatigues easily; his bladder cannot hold urine; his head cannot hold hair; and his mind has difficulty remembering. The quality of energy that holds things together (*chi*) is depleted, wih emphasis on the KIDNEY CHI. In *Selenium* one sees the first signs of DEFICIENT JING, the deepest level of *kidney* energy. In the next remedy we will discuss DEFICIENT JING.

We don't want to give the impression that *Selenium*, as a homeopathic or trace element, is "the remedy" for impotence or aging. In fact, there are many homeopathic remedies that the physician would study after taking a complete case, and there are many other vitamins or trace elements that might be necessary.

Baryta Carbonica: **Barium Carbonate**

Barium carbonate ($BaCO_3$) is a white, odorless, and tasteless powder. In nature it is found in the mineral whitherite, which forms large white crystals. All soluble compounds of *Baryta* are poisonous; a fatal dose is around 1 gram. *Baryta* is a muscle stimulant, particularly toxic to the heart since it causes violent palpitations or ventricular fibrillation. The homeopathic remedy, *Baryta Carbonica*, can be used for such symptoms if the total picture fits. Barium carbonate (*Baryta*) is not used in conventional medicine, but Barium sulphate is prepared as a chalk-like drink for the purpose of x-raying the intestine.

Barium, calcium, and strontium are closely related, classified in the periodic chart as alkaline earth metals. *Baryta* is the heaviest and least volatile of these, and the words "*Baryta*" and "*Barium*" are in fact derived from the Greek word for "heavy." It is the mass of the barium atom that makes it useful in x-ray technology because the rays are reflected by the large atom, revealing an opaque intestine. The pure metal was isolated in 1808 by Humphrey Davies. Commercially, barium carbonate is used as a flux in ceramics and as an ingredient in optical glass and fine glassware, but its most important use is in the production of permanent magnets used in loud-speakers.

Characteristics and Keynotes

In medicine, *Baryta Carbonia* is only used in homeopathy. Because of Dr. Hahnemann's unique method of converting insoluble metals into medicines, this mineral plays a role in homeopathic medicine. Like *Alumina* and other metals, *Baryta Carbonica* is prepared by trituration (see *Stannum*). *Baryta Carbonica* is employed against problems of old age or to treat underdeveloped

children. In either case, the *Baryta Carbonica* patient is mentally
backward, physically weak and possibly dwarfish in stature with
a poor memory, a timid personality, exhibiting childish or senile
behavior, and a great sensitivity to cold. *Baryta* is a deep and long-
acting remedy.

- Glands around the ears are swollen and painful; swollen ton-
  sils, inability to swallow anything but liquids; diseases of old
  men such as hardness of the testicles and prostate.
- Dwarfish, hysterical old women with deficient heat.
- Impotency, chronic dry cough, fetid food smells.
- Troubled sleep.
- Worse: when thinking of symptoms, washing, lying on the
  painful side; after meals.
- Better: when walking in the open air; when alone; after con-
  suming cold food.

Baryta, as can be seen from the above symptoms, is a very
peculiar and specific remedy, with a remarkable potential as a
healing agent.

Chinese Diagnosis

Baryta Carbonica is another wonderful example of a homeopathic remedy which presents a clear picture from a Chinese
perspective. In this case, *Baryta* matches the Chinese description
of a DEFICIENT JING disharmony. *Jing* is an enormously important phenomenon in the Oriental perspective of the bodily land-
scape. *Jing*, closely related to the *kidney* energy, is the essence of
life, but it should not be only equated with sperm or ova as these
are encompassed by the *jing*. *Jing* is the deepest aspect of the *yin*
essence of the body; it is nutritive and supportive. The *kidneys*
are said to store the *jing* and therefore are the root of the *zangfu*,
(the twelve organs). *Jing* is responsible for reproduction, growth,
ripening, and withering, and is related to the seven- and eight-
year cycles of life.[42]

Jing is partially derived from our parents. We are said to be
born with certain amounts of *jing* that we should not waste, since

it is an unrenewable resource. It can be restored by esoteric Taoist methods such as breathing and meditative techniques, but this is very difficult. Those who deplete their *jing* through an unhealthy lifestyle will have diminished the quality and length of their life. The most extreme signs of deficient *jing* are seen in the senile aged, and from an Oriental perspective the quality of *jing* explains why some people live to a hearty old age, and why others decline sooner. The symptoms of DEFICIENT JING are remarkably similar to those found in *Baryta Carbonica*, such as improper maturation and development, premature aging and senility, poor memory, brittle bones, falling hair and sexual weakness.[43] In DEFICIENT JING patterns, deeper than *Kidney yin* or *yang*, one sees evidence of grave deficiency. In Oriental medicine the *Kidneys* are said to rule the brain, called the "sea of marrow," and when the *kidneys* weaken, memory and concentration diminish. In Alzheimer's disease there are obvious signs of DEFICIENT JING. What factors lead to a premature deterioration of *jing*? Sexual excesses, devitalized diet, abuse of recreational or medical drugs, prolonged grief or fear are all possible factors, but one must also examine the parents and grandparents for clues to the origin of this deficiency. Chinese herbs like *rehmanniae* and *polygoni multiflori*, which build the *kidneys* and *blood*, can support the *jing*, as well as specific exercises and foods.

Thus concludes our discussion of remedy pictures. There are other remedies and patterns of disharmony that we would have liked to discuss, but we have at least enumerated a broad spectrum of Chinese energetic disharmonies and homeopathic remedies. The range of disharmony patterns we presented is quite comprehensive; it includes a majority of the main patterns found in Chinese medicine, and affords the reader a wide perspective of Chinese medical disharmonies. The remedies, though only a small portion of the homeopathic pharmacopoeia, are an excellent introduction to the world of homeopathic therapeutics. We hope the reader has found this section as interesting as it was for us to compile it.

8

Conclusions:
New Directions

Solvae et coagulae: to dissolve and reform.
a famous alchemical saying

As we discovered in our early years of training, there is an immense gap between theory and practice. After completing regular university curricula, we studied acupuncture for three years, and once we finished all those years of largely theoretical training, we thought we were very wise. In our first year of clinical practice, we were rudely exposed to the magnitude of our ignorance. Confronted with the complexities and contradictions of real, suffering people, our valiant theories lacked the foundation of experience; like many beginners, however, our lack of experience was compensated by enthusiasm and hard work. We truly loved this Oriental healing art with its delicate nuances and subtle philosophy. We had experienced how it could help people—our friends, our families, and ourselves—and we were eager to share the pragmatic healing art with others. Oriental medicine clearly had a role to play in American health care.

There were other obstacles to our goal. When we first started to practice, acupuncture was still considered an Oriental oddity, and few Americans realized its practical value. At that time few people recognized that acupuncture appears almost custom-made for fast-paced American life. With its ability to ease pain gently and induce relaxation without side effects or danger, the potential of acupuncture is being discovered throughout the Western world. But when we began our studies of Oriental medicine, we

225

were considered odd for embarking on such a career. How could two college-educated Americans abandon their successful careers? How could they begin a precarious adventure in a strange Oriental healing art that involved sticking needles into people! In this age of scientific medicine and technology, could this system have any real credibility? At that time acupuncture had almost no legal standing in the United States. Twelve years later, in 1988, the situation has changed dramatically. In the past decade we have witnessed a remarkable increase in public interest and knowledge about acupuncture, and currently it is being accepted and integrated into many spheres of American life.

As Westerners, we also experienced many cultural difficulties in our own study of acupuncture. Despite our enthusiasm for Oriental ideas, we initially approached our studies from a Western point of view. Even now, many years later, this bias still remains, though to a far lesser degree. There was much we would have to unlearn, and much we would absorb from protracted experience. As we have discussed, the circular model of the Orient is very different from the linear model of the West. Westerners, especially those with allopathic medical training, initially find Oriental medicine incomprehensible, naive, and even ridiculous. There were times when we shared these and many other critical ideas. The Western medical approach seems very logical, solid, and definite. One looks into a microscope or studies a chart and finds clear proof of disease, and on this level everything is clear and demonstrable.

In the initial stages of studying Oriental medicine everything is murky and unclear. What is *chi;* what are stagnation and deficiency; how can one possibly understand DEFICIENT KIDNEY YIN or DAMP SPLEEN? It requires a sympathy with the basic concepts, and a readiness to test and experience, to surmount this initial conceptual barrier. To fully understand the principles of Oriental medicine it is necessary to advance beyond theory. It is essential that the student is guided in the clinic and is told by the experienced doctor: Feel this pulse; this is a wiry *liver* pulse. See that tongue, the puffy shape, the yellow coated center; these signs indicate DAMP HEAT in the middle warmer. One can logically explain *chi* or microdoses until one is blue in the face and still reach no understanding. Oriental medicine and homeopathy are human sciences, based on bioenergetics and a careful scrutiny of people. Probably the most challenging part of our training was this task of making concepts like disharmony "patterns" come to life.

With each passing year of clinical experience, we develop more understanding. The disharmony patterns have become more recognizable, more discernible in people; they have become familiar, like friends. We understand their fine points, idiosyncrasies and quirks, as well as comprehending the larger picture. They have become a marvelous mirror into humanity, into the wide spectrum of health and disease, and in fact, something of great value has developed: a consistent ability to discern these patterns and to treat people successfully.

These patterns of disharmony are universal. We see disease not as an isolated factor in the body, but as an interconnection of physical, emotional, and mental qualities. People throughout history, of any race or culture, express disharmony patterns in the same way. An African, a Norwegian, and a Spaniard can all manifest clear signs of LIVER YANG RISING, with such symptoms as splitting headache, irritability, and impatience, or they can display the signs of *Nux Vomica* and benefit from taking this remedy. These patterns existed in ancient China two thousand years ago, and they will continue to exist in twenty-first century America. It is a source of great satisfaction to see our developing understanding of these patterns because it increases our ability to help people.

A nervous young man comes into the office complaining of insomnia, headaches, and fatigue. He has seen a regular physician and has received a variety of sleeping pills and anti-depressants, all to no avail—in fact, he feels worse. He is a thin muscular man with small dark shadows in the corners of his eyes. He finds it difficult to sit still. His tongue is quite thin and pointed with a distinct red tip; his pulse is thin and wiry, especially in the *kidney* position. At night he has difficulty going to sleep, his head churning with thoughts; in the late morning he wakes up, exhausted. The sleeping pills helped him for several weeks but made him drowsy during the day, and after a while he developed headaches on the top of his head. This man is suffering from DEFICIENT KIDNEY YIN. The lack of KIDNEY YIN or "water" has affected his *liver* and *heart*, producing anxiety and restlessness. One can alleviate this condition in a few treatments with acupuncture and herbs. Naturally, one must also examine the patient's diet and lifestyle and advise on any necessary adjustments. If one is thinking homeopathically, several remedies come to mind. In both systems one does not treat the insomnia *per se*, but rather the underlying disharmony that produces insomnia as one of its primary symptoms. Other insomniacs might require quite different treatment approaches.

Let us look at another patient, a quiet, soft-spoken young woman who complains of abdominal pains and an inability to lose weight. Lower G.I. series and other tests have revealed no pathology. She has a round, kindly face with a pale smooth complexion, and a soft, extremely moist, flabby tongue with a hint of purple in the middle. Her pulse is slow, deep and slippery, her movements are slow, and her voice is melodious. All her complaints are worse in cold damp weather. Clearly she is DEFICIENT SPLEEN and KIDNEY FIRE, a *damp* type person. Her middle warmer, particularly *spleen* and *stomach*, is lacking in transformative fire; therefore, her ability to convert food into energy is weakened. On inquiry she reveals that her diet has been completely inadequate for many years. She is completely surprised by this fact, exclaiming that no one—and certainly not her doctor!—had told her otherwise. Like many Americans her diet is extremely *yin*, lacking in vitality and energy; she eats a predominance of cold foods, such as salads, cold cuts, white bread, low-calorie refrigerated pop drinks and ice cream, and never varies her diet through the seasons. Her dietary habits exaggerate her basic constitutional weaknesses. Her mother also fought an endless battle against obesity, and later in life developed crippling arthritis in the hands and knees. There are several ways one would help this woman: dietary changes, acupuncture with moxabustion, and tonifying herbal blends to strengthen her *stomach/spleen*. From a homeopathic perspective one would find the most similar remedy. She is a *Calcarea* type, and will benefit greatly from taking this remedy at the right time.

Clinical Applications

Though we might give the impression that the application of these systems is easy, it most definitely is not. Homeopathy and Oriental medicine are disciplines based on laws and principles that take years to learn and fully absorb. Like the concert pianist or nuclear physicist, the student of these medical principles does not develop his talents overnight; his skill requires years of arduous preparation and training. Yeh Tien Shih, a famous Chinese physician, began studying medicine as a boy, first with his father, then with a Dr. Chu.[1] Initially, he simply followed Chu and watched him collect and prepare medicines. For several years the doctor did not speak much about medicine to Shih. Shih carried the old doctor's bag and perfomed menial tasks, like preparing fires, until the day when the doctor began to divulge his secrets; even at that stage in his education, it was several years before Shih was allowed to treat the simplest conditions.

Each of these two bioenergetic systems is like a fine craft in its love for detail, like a science in its large body of acquired knowledge, and like an art in its vision of integrating different parts. These sciences are based on living people; they are not derived from idle speculation or empty analysis. Dr. Hahnemann, for example, proved the first homeopathic drugs on himself, and in this way gained direct information about the use and efficacy of his remedies. The good holistic doctor observes and listens carefully, and from this information he sees a pattern. This ability requires years of consistent clinical practice, but for the great doctors the act seems effortless. There are countless stories in homeopathic and Oriental literature about the master who astounds his clients and pupils with his insight and healing success. Without wasting much time, he knows the remedy. Patients come to him from all corners; many have seen all the specialists; some of them have been given up as lost causes. A holistic master has the ability to penetrate to the core of the problem, to see the outline of disharmony, and, of course, to prescribe the correct treatment. But he has paid a steep price for this gift.

In the previous chapter we discussed in some detail the disharmony patterns of homeopathy and Chinese medicine, but we did not mean to imply that these two systems are interchangeable. In fact, any blending of these two systems must be approached with caution, even skepticism, as each system takes years to study and master. To utilize them both is a complex undertaking requiring years of research and work; there are no short-cuts in applying these systems, either alone or together.

In any case, why should a student of holistic medicine work with both of these systems? One would think that each by itself would be sufficient. However, there are limitations in any medical system, and in this case the potentials of synthesis are intriguing, to say the least.

The authors, trained as acupuncturists, recognize the broad, eight-branched base of Chinese medicine. Acupuncture can be effectively used by itself, but its efficacy is improved when combined with the eight branches, particularly herbal therapeutics, an internal medicine. However, we chose to work with homeopathy rather than Chinese herbology for several reasons. Though extremely effective, Chinese herbology has several practical limitations: the medicines come from far away; a convenient pharmacy is often hard to find; and the herbs are very expensive when compared to homeopathic remedies. Furthermore, homeopathic remedies are far easier to administer. Chinese medicines often have to be repeated once or twice a day for weeks or months, and the herbal teas have to be cooked up and often have a peculiar taste. Children, for example, are much more amenable to the homeopathic remedies; in fact, they love them! Homeopathy is also far easier to administer to elderly people, to animals, and to the chronically ill. Cats, for instance, are not too fond of acupuncture or herbal teas! Another advantage to homeopathy is that it has some modern clinical applications, such as the use of nosodes (remedies prepared from diseased tissue), which are not found in Chinese medicine.

The synthesis of homeopathy and acupuncture, however, is a challenging one; at this point, the authors use homeopathy primarily as an adjunct therapy for acute and chronic prescribing. The combined use of acupuncture and homeopathy in acute conditions such as colds, fevers, sprained ankles, shoulder and back pain, and other short-term problems is straightforward and effective. For example, a long-distance runner comes in complaining of a wrenched achilles tendon; in a week she has an important race which she must not miss. In an instance like this, the combined use of acupuncture and homeopathy is especially effective and will reduce the amount of treatments necessary to catalyze the healing. For acute back pain, remedies such as *Rhus Tox*, *Sulphur*, or *Ruta* can be selected and administered in low-potency doses, along with one or two acupuncture treatments combining moxabustion, acupuncture, and cupping (a specialized form of massage using glass suction cups). The acupuncturist can send his patient home with a vial of *Ruta Graveolens*, knowing that this remedy has a special efficacy for healing torn tendons. His work will be more efficient, effective, and not as costly for the patient.

Chronic and constitutional prescribing, however, is far more complex and requires both detailed knowledge and extensive clinical experience. Obviously, each of these systems requires years of study and experience. We have seen acupuncturists with a meager training in homeopathy suddenly prescribing remedies with wild abandon; likewise, we have seen medical doctors performing acupuncture after a weekend seminar. Many "classical" homeopaths are skeptical about introducing any form of therapy, even a bioenergetic system like acupuncture, during the course of homeopathic constitutional treatments. How will one know which modality is working? How will one measure the responses of the patient? Will the acupuncture alter the action of the homeopathic remedy? These and other arguments raise important questions about mixing these two distinct bioenergetic therapies. Since this kind of combined therapy is very new, the answers will not come soon. In our clinical experience each case must be approached differently: in some just acupuncture is sufficient; in others, homeopathy is more appropriate; and for still other cases, the two modalities can be used together with great success. A future book will address this subject in greater detail.

Currently, there is an innovative synthesis of acupuncture and homeopathy in the use of sophisticated electronic instruments that provide diagnosis and treatment. This application has largely come out of Germany where a group of doctors, led by Rheinhold Voll, have been using electronic devices to diagnose and treat for several decades. These devices are founded upon the electromagnetic fields of the body and the acupuncture points and meridians. The instruments measure tiny degrees of bioelectric resistance at acupuncture test points. On a meter these instruments can depict organ weakness, excess, and degeneration, with a precision and clarity that caters to the scientist in all of us. Furthermore, treatment can be administered using tiny electrical currents generated by the instrument. Perhaps the most controversial application of these devices is their use in testing vitamins, herbs, drugs, and homeopathics for treatment. A common clinical application is to test different homeopathic remedies to see which one balances the reading on the meter; in this way remedies are often selected.

The authors have had limited experience with these devices and regard them with cautious respect. They offer a valid new application for acupuncture and homeopathy, and no doubt they will increase in popularity in this age of electronic technology and love of devices in general. But, one must ask, will they become barriers between patient and doctor; will they reduce the doctor's own abilities to observe and diagnose; and will they result in allopathic-like prescribing of homeopathics? Ultimately, and we say this with great emphasis, the human organism is and will remain the finest diagnostic instrument ever devised, and—as demonstrated by the great acupuncturists and homeopaths from the past and present—the sensory, mental, and intuitive abilities of man can be remarkable.

Comparisons and Contrasts

In Chapter Seven we briefly discussed the idea of remedy types and described how this concept exists in both systems. In homeopathy we saw the *Nux Vomica* or *Lycopodium* types; in Chinese medicine we saw the LIVER YANG or KIDNEY DEFICIENT types. Each person might become ill in a unique way, but each has something in common with others. The Chinese doctor will not treat every case of LIVER YANG RISING in the same way, because in each individual there are fine details and nuances that he must not overlook. However, for each LIVER YANG patient his treatments will, for the most part, follow a similar pattern. Certain people are susceptible to LIVER YANG symptoms, while others will never have such complaints. When you tell an Oriental doctor that your good friend is a LIVER YANG type, he will smile knowingly, perhaps with a little sympathy, because he will know that your friend is impulsive and hot-headed. The LIVER YANG type is also outgoing and energetic, and in "normal" conditions he is a very favorable type of person. These different types of individual are a fundamental fact in holistic prescribing. Each type has general characteristics and predispositions. The *Nux Vomica* type is very different from the *Calcarea*, and generally he will heal faster. The *Nux Vomica* type might need other remedies in certain cases, but these remedies all tend to have some relation to *Nux*.

The understanding of types is a holistic perspective derived from careful observation of people, not in parts, but in unity. Properly understood, this process does not lead to stereotyping. The holistic doctor studies each person as an individual, but always sees the relation of the individual to others of similar type. When the patient comes in complaining of headaches, he studies the whole person, not just the headache. He wants to know all the specifics of the headache; where it is; when it is worse or better; and he wants to know about the lungs, the kidneys, the sleep, the habits, and all the other pertinent facts about this person. If necessary, he wants to have blood tests, x-rays, and CAT scans. In this way the doctor begins to gain an understanding of the totality of the patient and thus forms a disharmony pattern. The best doctors of any school study the generals and the specifics, for this is the essence of good doctoring.

Throughout this book we have emphasized the similarities between these two systems. There are, in fact, major differences, some that we have completely ignored until now. We'd like to broaden the picture and discuss some of these differences as well as some similarities that we have not broached. In response to the inevitable question, "Which system is better?" we cannot say. Both have their advantages and limitations; with certain people in a specific setting, one or the other might be better. Generally, however, we would not select one system over the other.

Chinese medicine is based on an ancient cosmology that touches all corners of life. It is a unitary vision of man within the cosmos of society and nature. The Taoist concepts of *yin* and *yang* permeate all phases of life, not just medicine, and the true Chinese doctor—an ideal difficult to find—is skilled in acupuncture, herbs, dietary consultation, and other related subjects. He might also teach meditation, T'ai Chi, or other exercises. If trained in Western medicine, he might also perscribe allopathic drugs.

Oriental doctors use herbal formulas, needles, their hands and many other tools. Acupuncture, for example, can work directly with the body, its energies, muscles, and bones, and in this way effect profound changes. Homeopaths, on the other hand, primarily use potentized remedies. They are blessed with an elegant and uncluttered system of medicine which is methodical and practical, yet sophisticated and philosophical. Usually trained in biochemical medicine, homeopaths must also have an extensive knowledge of hundreds of remedies. Homeopathic pharmacists are probably the most exacting in the world, and extremely concerned about the purity of their medicines. The process of manufacturing these remedies requires the utmost cleanliness, precision, and care to ensure the purity of the final product. Oriental medicine is more earthy and less exacting, but the Oriental doctor must have an expansive knowledge of hundreds of herbs and acupuncture points. A Chinese pharmacist must be a walking encyclopedia, not only on the identification and action of hundreds of healing substances, but also on the variations of preparation and administration. Chinese herbal formulas are carefully blended to fit the imbalance of the individual, and therefore must be prepared and prescribed with care and skill.

Both systems utilize the vast storehouse of nature's potential healing agents prepared from plant, mineral, animal and insect products. People ignorant of the energetic basis of Chinese herbs think it a curious hodge-podge of bizarre superstition. On the contrary, each remedy has been studied and tested for centuries. Each remedy is known to have a specific energetic action according to *yin/yang* and the five phases, and each is known to have a complementary or antagonistic relationship with other remedies. Homeopaths also use many bizarre substances to create their remedies. Both systems make remedies from snake venom; both utilize toxic plants like deadly nightshade and monkshood, as well as common garden herbs like sage, dandelion and comfrey. Both disciplines utilize minerals like oyster shell and sulphur, but each employs its own unique methods of preparation. It is important to remember that in Chinese herbal medicine the remedy is prepared directly from the crude substance, be it root, seed, or mineral, whereas in homeopathy the crude substance is converted into a potentized remedy by repeated dilution and succussion.

The healing action of their respective remedies is quite different. Let us use as an example, a strange remedy prepared from the common toad, *Bufo rana*. In homeopathy *Bufo* is a minor remedy used for epilepsy with specific symptoms, and for people obsessed with sex and prone to excess masturbation. Apparently this remedy, prepared from the glandular secretion of the toad, is used by certain tribes in the Amazon where the women diminish their husband's lust with the extract.[2] The toad secretion is known to have a strong effect on the central nervous system; when injected into rats, it can cause strong convulsions,[3] confirming its use by homeopaths in treating certain kinds of epileptic convulsions. In China, the secretion has been used for centuries. Its energetic actions are cooling and detoxifying, and eradicate summer heat and dampness. Recent research has demonstrated that sterol derivatives of the secretion have an anti-inflammatory effect, which verifies its use by herbal healers.[4] It is interesting to note that one of the herbal uses of *Bufo rana* is as a treatment for a sudden loss of consciousness caused by summer heat stroke— reflective again of its homeopathic use in treating convulsions. Therefore, each system uses the remedy in its own way, but there is some overlap in usage. Another important similarity is that both systems use the complete substance, unlike biochemical medicine which only isolates the most potent molecules. These two systems inherently understand the unique healing power of the whole in which there is a particular design.

In addition, each system teaches a respect for the knowledge of modern medical research and technology. Homeopaths are, for the most part, trained as medical doctors. Many Oriental doctors are trained in Western medicine, and those who are not generally have a basic understanding of modern medicine. One does not have to use chemical drugs to be a good doctor, but one must have a good understanding of anatomy and physiology.

The Chinese doctor is well trained in "reading" the signs of the body, a skill surpassing his homeopathic or allopathic colleagues. For him, the external body is a book that can reveal many secrets. Ears, tongue, pulse, complexion, birth marks, posture are part of the language of the body; he interprets them all with a subtlety that boggles the Western mind. For example, a Chinese doctor who is properly trained in the ancient art of reading the face can use facial clues in reaching a diagnosis about a patient's character and health. Like all inductive sciences, this skill requires a mixture of facts, intuition, and an ability spontaneously to sense the underlying pattern. The good practitioner is also aware of the limitations of the system, and he does not rely on this one facet for diagnosis. He will also study the patient's medical history, pulse and tongue. Different parts of the face reflect different organs or parts of the body. One studies such details as the basic shape of the head; the shape of the lips and nose; the width, density, and shape of eyebrows; and the special marks of coloring of the skin;

all have an inner significance. The ancient axion, "As above, so below," is applied to every facet of Chinese medicine.

The Oriental doctor also understands the flow of energy through the organs and meridians, and the specific location of any pain can be significant. For example, a pain on the outer aspect of the thigh might involve the gall bladder meridian and its energetic functions. This can be very valuable information for the practitioner and patient, for other practitioners might spend months fruitlessly trying to relieve this pain in the thigh with no knowledge of the larger picture. In our practice we have seen this countless times with patients suffering from pinched nerves, migraines, sciatica, and a host of other problems.

The homeopath pays similar attention to detail in studying the patient, but his goal is to use the accumulated facts to find the best remedy. For diagnosis and treatment he might use other methods (blood test or nutrition, for example), but his basic tool is homeopathy. Each system, in its own way, "reads" the whole person, and then derives a picture or pattern of disharmony. In both systems, determination of these patterns rely to a great extent on the study of modalities: how a person responds to the environment, including weather, time of day, seasons, and emotions. Modalities are critical to the proper discernment of disharmony patterns.

These patterns, however, are based on different methodological languages. While homeopathy is grounded in the law of similars, Oriental medicine is based on the laws of *yin* and *yang*. The homeopathic remedy does not heal by imparting any new power or quality to the tissue, but by stimulating the inherent healing power. Homeopathic remedies are essentially quantum packets of bioenergetic information which effect the whole person. Chinese medicine is based on the principle of *yin/yang*. Both herbal and acupuncture treatments work on a physical level—like vitamins and biochemicals—and on an energetic level. Anyone who has had experience with acupuncture knows that it can directly affect the tissue by relaxing the local muscle tension and stimulating circulation of blood, but at the same time stimulating the bioelectrical energy. The same is true for herbs. Chinese herbal formulas can sustain the body in different ways; they can also balance and manipulate the energy. Ginseng, for example, is nourishing as it contains vitamins and calories, but also builds the energy of the *spleen* and *stomach* (it is said to enter those meridians).

Chinese medicine, like homeopathy, heals on several different levels, but does so by abiding by the principles of *yin*, *yang*, and balance. Chinese medicine uses the principles of tonification and sedation. If a patient is deficient KIDNEY YANG with many cold signs, low back pain, chilliness, and impotence, the physician might apply heat (moxa) to specific *kidney* points. This is what we mean by "tonification." Sedation techniques would be used in excess, *yang* conditions, such as a pounding headache.

Contrary to allopathic practice, both systems encourage the domestic use of natural remedies as well as the idea of medical self-reliance. Orientals have employed herbs and home remedies for centuries, and many common folk are adept at curing simple ailments. Homeopathy also has a highly-effective home and first-aid application. The remedies are totally safe, easy to use, and superb for disease prevention. We have both used homeopathic first-aid kits for a wide variety of ailments. Incidentally, these remedies are wonderful for children and pets because they are safe and can be administered easily. Children never object to the little homeopathic pellets, and because their energy is less cluttered, they respond faster than adults. Louis' old golden retriever, Simba, was greatly relieved of crippling arthritis by homeopathic and acupuncture treatments.

Although their methods are different, both systems are preventative in orientation, and subscribe to the idea that a healthy body will repel most illness. Many aspects of Oriental medicine are directly used to maintain health; T'ai Chi (exercises), dietary practices, and yoga are good examples. Dietary practice is an integral part of Oriental medicine and very valuable as it is based on *yin/yang* and the five phases. Like Hippocrates, the Chinese follow the adage that food is the best medicine, the first line of defense. All foods are classified in varying degrees of *yin* and *yang*, and according to the five phases; in this way diet can be altered to suit a particular disharmony. In China there are marvelous restaurants where one is diagnosed by a doctor—not a waiter— and then served a dinner according to one's disharmony pattern! Homeopaths do not use dietary change as much as their Eastern colleagues, but they do use dietary facts to help determine the remedy.

According to some accounts, doctors in ancient China were paid to keep their patients healthy. If a client became sick, his doctor would have to pay for the expenses of restoring health. How different this is from today's health care system! Even if this story is a legend, its very existence points to a very different philosophy of healing.

As for more direct methods of treatments, homeopaths pre- dated their allopathic colleagues with measures against infectious diseases. Dr. Swann, a homeopath, prepared a dose of *Tuber- culinum* from tuberculosis sputum in 1871, several decades before the scientist Koch introduced a similar procedure to the world.[6] Homeopaths also prepared *Lyssin* from the saliva of a mad dog before Louis Pasteur made this technique famous.[7] Another in- teresting fact is that homeopaths also used preparations of gold, digitalis, selenium, and nitroglycerine before they were introduced to regular medicine. There is no mention of these facts in the stan- dard medical texts.

Homeopathy is most sophisticated in its use of nosodes for treatment. *Tubercullinum*, mentioned above, is a major constitu- tional remedy, not used to cure tuberculosis, but for those who resonate with its broad symptomatology. These nosodes are im- portant additions to the homeopathic materia medica and find ready application in chronic prescribing. They offer a type of treat- ment approach not available in Chinese medicine.

In terms of diagnosis, homeopaths are very thorough in the depth and complexity of their casetaking, and in their understand- ing of the interrelation of psyche and body. More than their Orien- tal colleagues, they delve into the emotions and mind; in China today there is a distinct somatic and pragmatic orientation to the practice of acupuncture and herbal medicine, whereas in America and Europe Oriental medicine is often influenced by a more eclectic and psychological approach. Acupuncture, therefore, is developing along different lines in America, and many of the acupuncturists (such as the authors) have a broad training in Eastern and Western ideas and practices.

In the previous chapter the reader was introduced to such multi-dimensional remedies as *Lachesis* and *Calcarea*, where one sees the relationship between the psyche and body in all its complexity. *Lycopodium*, a great remedy for weak liver and digestion, is a classic personality portrait of cowardice. Homeopathy, like Chinese medicine, heals problems of the mind and heart, and when psychological therapy is necessary, it is a great adjunct. We have seen both systems work well in cases of substance abuse, depression, anxiety, post-accident trauma, shock, and other related problems. In this kind of therapy there is no chance of chemical dependence; side effects are very rare; and the integrity of the whole person is respected.

Because these systems work with the natural healing power of the body, and because the goal is to create balance with the minimum intervention, they are both safe and gentle systems. Underlying their medical practice is a profound respect for the ecological and bioenergetic relationships in man and nature. As Western civilization inundates herself with pollutants in the water, air, earth and food, this increases the potential for large scale health problems. The same disregard for the external environment is reflected in the pollution of the internal ecology of body and mind. The Western diet is flooded with stimulants like sugar, coffee and recreational drugs, and with devitalized refined food. In addition, the body is permeated with powerful medical drugs; all are flooding the body in a way that has never occurred on this planet. For instance, the average American consumes one hundred and twenty pounds of sugar a year, compared to seven pounds eighty years ago. Furthermore, what of the subtle, long-term effect of powerful medications now taken every day by millions of people? The long-term abuse of penicillin, for example, is barely questioned.[8]

What is the price people will pay? The body, like the external environment, is a resilient ecosystem, but it has its limits. The sum of all these pollutants must eventually disturb its homeostasis and overtax the liver and kidneys, and the nervous and immune systems. And, indeed, there is growing and ominous evidence of profound changes in the health of people in industrialized countries, such as an increase in so-called "allergies," immune-deficiency diseases and cancer.

Modern man at times displays a hostile attitude towards the inner and outer environments. In lifestyle and health he has a preference for short-term stimulation and effect. These two bio-energetic systems represent a deeper feeling towards life; they are part of a movement towards an understanding of the complex web of relationships in nature. Through technology and science we have learned to control our environment, truly a great gift, but this direction has become excessive, perhaps based on fear and greed. There has to be a balance between human beings and the natural world to which they belong, a relation based on a sensitivity for the sacred gift of life. For the past two hundred years science has created a bleak vision of man, nature, and the earth, a sterile, mechanical model that opposed the emotionalism of the middle ages. Nowadays, however, both new and ancient influences are permeating science, and the potential for positive change are great. Twenty years ago ecology was a minor issue relegated to crackpots and eccentric scientists; now it is a major public issue facing all of us. As human beings we are an integral part of the flux of life on this planet, an individual cell in a much larger organism. This ecological and holistic model has yet to be fully understood in Western medicine. Chinese medicine and homeopathy fill this gaping hole by applying the natural laws of healing.

Medicine and Beyond

Before concluding this book we would also like to acknowledge other great holistic systems that still exist on this planet. In India there is the ancient, venerable Ayurvedic medicine, closely intertwined with spiritual life and the Sanskrit texts. Though Tibetan civilization was decimated by the Communist Chinese, its medicine still survives, with even a few Tibetan doctors residing in America. Tibetan medicine, highly spiritual in essence, is a fascinating blend of Ayurvedic, Chinese, and Tibetan ideas and practices. And we must not neglect the rich heritage of the American Indians whose medicine was imbued with a holistic understanding of man and his relationship to nature. There are also many bioenergetic therapies that have arisen in recent time, all of which reflect an understanding of the primacy of bioenergy in health. Some of these include Reichian therapy, polarity therapy, osteopathy, radionics, Bach flower remedies, certain transpersonal therapies, and others.

There are many approaches to healing, and they all have their strengths and limitations. Modern biochemical medicine has made some great advances, especially in emergency cases, surgery, and the treatment of infectious diseases, and we certainly would be reluctant to return to "simpler" eras. Although one of the most valid criticisms of this approach is its overreliance on technology and quantification—the patient becomes an object to be measured and tested—many modern doctors nevertheless display a broadminded perspective and caring attitude towards the individual. There is an impeccable attention toward the patient that is perhaps the most important quality of healing—something that any doctor of any system can demonstrate.

One important fact that we have neglected is that holistic medicine is too often a fuzzy concept, with all the pitfalls and contradictions of a new cause. Because it is now an idea in vogue, all kinds of people are jumping on the wagon and making all sorts of preposterous claims, just because they give vitamins or have some clever electronic gadget. The approach of many "holistic practitioners" is vague and eclectic, not based on time-tested foundations of coherent ideas. Quite wrongly, holistic medicine has become a gigantic catch-all for alternative methods: liberal psychotherapists and doctors, chiropracters, nutritionists, acupuncturists, homeopaths, and many others. Practitioners who use noninvasive therapy like to call themselves "holistic" whether or not they are fully trained; such misrepresentation leads to a confused public image and lack of clear definition, and a dubious relation with conventional medicine.

We would like to make a clear distinction here: on one hand there is an eclectic holistic *approach,* and on the other there is a holistic *medicine* based on laws and principles such as those expounded in this book. Traditional Chinese medicine and homeopathy are two fine examples of holistic medicine. Holistic medicine is more than a caring attitude and a well-rounded approach; it is more than an understanding of the relationship between body, emotions, and mind. The word "holistic" infers a unitary force in the domain of body/mind. This unitary force is not a concept or symbol; it is the life energy of all living things. It has been recognized by all ancient holistic systems from around the world. And it ultimately accounts for the wholism denoted by the term "holistic," specifically as it relates to medicine and healing. Not only is it the living energy, it also is the basic regulating force in health, influencing bodily functions, emotions, and thoughts, and maintaining all in balance. A primary theme of this book has been that holistic medicine is a healing science based on bioenergetics. This medical therapy, as we pointed out in Chapters One and Two, is ancient and universal, and in certain cultures it has culminated in sophisticated systems such as acupuncture and homeopathy.

Hippocrates, considered the father of Western medicine, emphasized that the physician is the servant of nature, and that he must use as little intervention as possible in restoring health. He shall not force what can't be forced, nor must he be passive towards that which must be pushed. He must rely on gentle methods before relying on heroic measures. Hippocrates used food as his first line of defense against disease. Throughout history, doctors have been guilty in their overeagerness to conquer disease, and thus fall into the trap of doing too much. There are instances when this approach is unavoidable, but all too often it is the patient who suffers from these heroic measures. In the art of healing, the doctor must move with the delicacy of a bird in motion, yet have the potential power of a tiger.

Let us, once again, look at the words of health and disease. The English word "health" originates from the Sanskrit term connoting "wholeness" and "completeness." The unifying force, the bioenergy, gives life to the body/mind; it regulates health; it brings together the different parts. Dis-ease is a fragmenting, an imbalance, a breaking apart. The cancer cell is a fitting image of imbalance because it no longer knows its place in the kingdom of the body and forges its own path of destruction. The cancer cell is a fragment of cellular disorder that defies the unifying force of life. The balance of life has been so compromised, so disturbed, that the process of disorder takes hold and accelerates. The web of influence that integrates and preserves has been broken. Healing is a restoring of the integrity, but the question of health and disease is even larger than this.

Is the sole purpose of medicine to alleviate suffering and pain and to prolong the life of this body? Alternative and biochemical therapies are often directed towards the goal of making the body more comfortable—a fine goal to a certain level—but what is the role of this disease process? Is it simply due to accident of outside forces—bacteria, virus, evil spirits—or is there more that is invisible to our immediate perception? In ancient healing systems the physician tended not only to physical discomfort and illness; he was also a mediator between the person and the community and the higher forces in nature. In the modern world, however, there is no recognition of higher forces in nature. The balancing of health involves a relation of the individual to his inner and outer environment, and to the forces within the cosmos. We can offer no answers in this search, only more questions. Whom do we serve in this brief life span on this planet—our own physical needs and comforts? What is the purpose of this miraculous gift of life? These questions have been lost in modern practice. Too often the doctor is a specialist or a technician, oriented to symptoms of the physical body, whether he is an alternative or biochemical practitioner.

The health of the person involves the body, emotions, and mind as well as the spirit—the totality of each unique being. It also involves the person's connection to higher forces of nature, and ultimately to the mystery of life itself. In the ordinary sense, health is something that can be catalyzed by a doctor, but there is also an understanding that health must come from the individual. The doctor cannot force someone to live who wants to die, nor can he heal someone who refuses to accept the role disease plays in his life. Disease is "a breaking apart" which often involves a mental or emotional dissolution: a "dis-ease," a lesson to be absorbed, an attitude to be lost or gained. The person might be out of balance in some aspect of his life, such as his relation to self, occupation, or family. Healing involves a resolution on mental, social, and emotional levels, a domain that ultimately involves the person's own responsibility and personal growth. In the holistic model we see how the individual exists within the dynamic matrix of himself, family, society, nature, life energy, cosmic forces; and that healing can involve any or all of these levels.

In this book we have explored parallels between two great medical systems, seemingly separated by an abyss of culture and time. That they do share profound similarities is a remarkable validation of holistic theory and disharmony patterns, and a testimony to an alternative approach to medicine which challenges our Western assumptions about health and disease. This book, like many others, is calling for a new direction to medicine. Rather than "holistic," we prefer to call this direction "complementary medicine," a synthesis of biochemical and bioenergetic therapies that strive to work with the healing power of the body. We believe that the frontiers of medicine lie not with genetic engineering or organ transplants, but in a renewed exploration of the root of life, bioenergy. In the sixteenth century, when William Harvey proved that the blood circulated in the vessels, a giant step was taken in medicine. With the recognition and pursuit of bioenergy, there will be a quantum leap!

Notes

Chapter 1

1. S. Hahnemann, *The Organon of Medicine*, pp. 14–15.

2. See *The Web That Has No Weaver*, Chap. 2 for another, slightly different perspective on *chi*.

3. J. Needham, *Celestial Lancets*, p. 16.

4. Quoted in F. Mann, *Acupuncture: Cure of Many Diseases*, p. 55.

5. A. Carrell, *Man the Unknown*, p. 3.

6. T. Kaptchuk, Lecture notes, New England School of Acupuncture, 1982.

7. M. Porkert, "The Intellectual and Social Impulses Behind the Evolution of Traditional Chinese Medicine," *Asian Medical Systems*, p. 63.

8. This quote is from the immortal *Tao Teh Ching*, a Taoist book by Lao Tse.

9. R. Siu, *Chi: A Neo-Taoist Approach*, p. 27.

10. Quoted in R. De Ropp, *The New Prometheans*, p. 89.

11. "Interview: Rupert Sheldrake, Ph.D.," *New Realities*, Vol. V, No. 5, 1983, pp. 8, 10–15.

12. H. Burr, *The Fields of Life*, p. 33.

13. This discussion of Newton is largely based on information from Fritjof Capra's *The Tao of Physics*, chap. 4.

14. D. Bohm, "On the Intuitive Understanding of Nonlocality as Implied by Quantum Theory," *Foundation of Physics*, Vol. 5, 1975, pp. 96, 102, cited in the *Tao of Physics*, p. 124.

15. L. Dossey, *Space, Time, and Medicine*, p. 146.

16. This debate is continuously being revived in articles as there seems no resolution in sight, and there is no definite evidence that we are "winning the war on cancer" despite incredible expenditures.

17. L. Dossey, op. cit., p. 8.

18. M. Lappé, *When Antibiotics Fail*.

19. J. Needham, *Science and Civilization in China*, Vol. 2, pp. 280–281. We are also indebted to T. Kaptchuk for clarifying the term "disharmony patterns."

Chapter 2

1. J. Houston, *The Possible Human*, p. XII.

2. C. Thakkur, *Ayurveda*, p. 4.

3. M. Coddington, *In Search of the Healing Energy*, p. 46.

4. I. Newton, *The Principa Mathematica*, p. 547.

5. C. Gillispie, *Dictionary of Scientific Biography*, p. 63.

6. R. Eaton, *Descartes Selection*, p. XIII.

7. Ibid., p. XXVI.

8. R. Grossinger, *Planet Medicine*, p. 208.

9. R. Becker, *The Body Electric*, p. 64.

10. C. Gillispie, *Concise Dictionary of Scientific Biography*, p. 581.

11. W. Mann, *Orgone, Reich, and Eros*, p. 100.

12. D. Price, *Science Since Babylonia*, pp. 84–89.

13. E. Russell, *Report on Radionics*, pp. 17–18.

14. E. Boirac, *Our Hidden Forces*, p. 89.

15. W. Mann, op. cit., p. 106.

16. H. Burr, *Blueprint For Immortality*, p. 127.

17. Ibid., 95.

18. W. Mann, op. cit., p. 106.

19. Ibid., p. 106.

20. Ibid., p. 106.

21. E. Russell, op. cit., p. 20.

22. S. Krippner, *The Kirlian Aura*, p. 136.

23. Ibid., p. 135.

24. R. Siu, *Chi: A Neo-Taoist Approach To Life*, p. 257.

25. R. Becker, op. cit., p. 70.

26. G. Taubes, "An Electrifying Possibility," *Discover:* 1986, April, Vol. 7, #4, p. 33.

27. Ibid., p. 25.

28. Ibid., pp. 25–26.

29. A. Lehninger, *Biochemistry*, p. 4.

30. D. Boorstin, *The Discoverers*, pp. 338–339.

31. G. Taubes, op. cit., p. 37.

32. R. Becker, op. cit., pp. 332, 347.

33. Ibid., p. 347.

34. E. Kueshana, *The Ultimate Frontier*, p. 260.

35. G. De la Warr, *New Worlds Beyond the Atom*, p. 152.

Chapter 3

1. W. Tiller quoted in the *Journal of Holistic Health*, 1978.

2. Gandhi quoted in the *World Homeopathic Directory* 1982 (New Delhi: World Homeopathic Links, 1982).

3. H. Coulter, *Divided Legacy*, V. III, pp. 288, 449, 467.

4. H. Selye, *The Stress of Life*, p. 83.

5. Ibid., p. 82.

6. J. Borysenko, 'Psychoimmunerology," *Revision Journal*, (Spring, 1984) p. 57.

7. H. Coulter, op. cit., Vol. II, p. 311 fn.

8. S Hahnemann, *Lesser Writings*, p. 512.

9. T. Bradford, *Life and Letters of Dr. Samuel Hahnemann*, p. 9.

10. G. Koehler, *The Handbook of Homeopathy*, p. 14.

11. H. Lu, *The Yellow Emperor's Classic of Internal Medicine and the Difficult Classic*, p. 484: In the paragraph where this quote is taken, the ancient Chinese writer acknowledges the law of similars and contraries.

12. L. Boyd, *The Study of the Simile in Medicine,* p. 9

13. Ibid., pp. 13, 14.

14. H. Coulter, *Homeopathic Science and Modern Medicine,* pp. 48–49. Dr. Coulter gives remarkable account of a reproving from the beginning of this century, conducted by a doctor for Boston University School of Medicine. Fifty "provers" were recruited from various cities, as well as host of specialists to conduct the proving. No one involved in the proving knew they were reproving *Belladonna.* The result was a study 665 pages long that completely verified the efficacy of the provings done in the nineteenth century.

15. Ibid., p. 35.

16. *The Patriotic Ledger,* Thursday, Nov. 14, 1985, p. 37: (Newspaper article).

17. A. Stebbing, "Hormesis—The Stimulation of Growth by Low Levels of Inhibitors," (1982) pp. 213–234: Also in Dana Ullman's *Monograph in Homeopathic Research.* Vol. II, Homeopathic Educational Services, Berkeley, Ca., 1986.

18. Ibid., p. 217.

19. J. Stephenson, "A Review of Investigations into the Action of Substances in Dilutions Greater than 1x 10–24 (Microcdilutions)," *Journal of American Institute of Homeopathy,* November, 1955, Vol. 48.

20. J. Stephenson and G. P. Barnard, "Fresh Evidence for a Biophysical Field," *Journal of the American Institute of Homeopathy,* April/May/June, 1969, Vol. 62. See Dana Ullman's Monograph Vol. 1.

21. H. Coulter, *Homeopathy and Modern Science,* p. 54.

22. A. Scofield, "Experimental Research in Homeopathy—A Critical Review." *British Homeopathic Journal,* 73, 3, 161–180 and July, 1984, 73, 4, September 1984, 211–226.

23. *Aspects of Research in Homeopathy,* Vol. 1–1983, Boiron, France.

24. S. Ries, "Triacontanol: A New Naturally Occurring Plant Growth Regulator," *Science,* 195, 4284, pp. 1339–1341.

25. R. Gibson, "Homeopathic Therapy in Rheumatoid Arthritis: Evaluation by Double-Blind Clinical Therapeutic Trial," *British Journal of Clinical Pharmacology,* May, 1980, 9, 453–459.

26. M. Shipley, "Controlled Trial of Homeopathic Treatment of Osteoarthritis," *Lancet,* 1983, pp. 97–98.

27. Scofield, op. cit., p. 162.

28. P. Flanagan, *Elixir of the Ageless*, p. 8.

29. G. Murchie, *The Seven Mysteries of Life*, pp. 449, 450.

30. P. Callinan, "The Mechanism of Action of Homeopathic Remedies— Towards a Definitive Model," *Journal of Complementary Medicine*, July, 1985, p. 45.

31. P. W. Bridgeman, *The Physics of High Pressure*, 1949.

32. From lectures and discussions with Marcel Vogel, scientist, in 1985.

33. P. Callinan, op. cit., p. 47.

34. P. Callinan, op. cit., pp. 48–52.

35. D. Reilly, "Is Homeopathy a Placebo Response? Controlled Trial of Homeopathic potency, with Pollen in Hayfever as Model," *The Lancet*, October 18, 1986, p. 885.

Chapter 4

1. D. Eisenberg, *Encounters with Qi*, p. 135.

2. H. Lu, *A Complete Translation of [The Nei Ching] The Yellow Emperor's Classic of Internal Medicine and The Difficult Classic*, p. 2.

3. J. Needham, *Celestial Lancets*, pp. 90–91.

4. J. Hassett, "Acupuncture is Proving its Points," *Psychology Today:* 1980, December, p. 81.

5. F. Mann, *Acupuncture: The Ancient Chinese Art of Healing*, p. v: This quote is from Aldous Huxley's forward for Dr. Mann's book.

6. Quoted from a lecture given by Dr. Pomeranz at the New England School of Acupuncture.

7. R. Becker, *The Body Electric*, pp. 233–236.

8. J. Darras, "Etude des méridiens d'acupuncture par les traceurs radioactifs," *Bull. Acad. Natle. Med.:* 1985, 169 n° 7 pp. 1071– 1075, Seance de 22 Octobre 1985.

9. G. Taubes, "An Electrifying Possibility," *Discover:* 1986, April Vol. 7 #4 p. 33.

10. B. Holbrook, *The Stone Monkey*, Chapter One. In this chapter ("The Terminal and Prerevolutionary Conditions of Western Sci-

ence") Yale anthropologist B. Holbrook thoroughly discusses this issue, especially the idea of technological pollution (from nuclear waste to chemotherapy production contributing to a rise in cancer rates).

11. N. Bohr, *Atomic Physics and the Description of Nature*, p. 2.

12. Throughout this book, Chinese diagnosis (a.k.a. patterns of disharmony) will be set in small (lower case) capitals to distinguish them from the Western terminology. Also, Chinese words, and words used in the Chinese sense or meaning, will be italicized: liver = Western sense, *liver* = Chinese sense.

13. V. Cobb, *Logic*, p. 61.

14. D. Loye, *The Sphinx and the Rainbow*, pp. 24–29.

15. P. Eckman, *Closing the Circle*, p. 16.

16. B. Lo, *The Essence of T'ai Chi Chu'uan*, p. 7.

17. J. Needham, *The Shorter Science and Civilization in China: 1*, pp. 50–53; D. Li, *The Ageless Chinese*, pp. 376–377.

18. J. Needham, op. cit., pp. 30–32.

19. J. Needham, *Celestial Lancets*, pp. 30–31.

20. P. Huard, *Chinese Medicine*, pp. 31–32.

21. H. Hsu, *Chen's History of Chinese Medical Science*, pp. 49–51.

22. P. Huard, op. cit., pp. 16–18 & H. Hsu, op. cit., pp. 20–23.

23. H. Hsu, op. cit., pp. 24–27.

24. Ibid., pp. 74–77.

25. Ibid., pp. 78–81.

26. Oriental medicine in modern China has been stripped of its Taoist esoteric origins and trappings. Of interest, too, is that Chinese acupuncture and herbal medicine are but one style practiced in the Orient. For example, Korea and Japan have distinctive styles of acupuncture. However, they all use a similar "vocabulary." It is also important to mention that there are different "schools" of Oriental medicine. Often there is a dichotomy between the *yin/yang* school, who tend to be herbally oriented, and the "five phase" school who tend to be acupuncturists. The "five phase school" is itself divided into several "camps." Is it any wonder that we chose to avoid

this confusion in our book? We tried to maintain a pluralistic perspective. The authors, though primarily trained in the Chinese *yin/yang* "school" (the eight principles), have studied other "schools," such as Japanese and Korean. In America today, acupuncture and herbalism, influenced by American culture and people, are following a new and distinct course.

Chapter 5

1. T. Kaptchuk, *The Web That Has No Weaver*, p. 15: Quoting from J. Needham, *Science and Civilization in China*, Vol. 1, pp. 280–281.

2. This quote is a well known Taoist teaching; it is paraphrased in H. Ni., *The Book of Changes and the Unchanging Truth*, p. 31, and is common throughout acupuncture texts.

3. O. Brunler, *Rays and Radiation*, p. 5–7.

4. R. Eaton, *Descartes Selections*, p. XXI.

5. H. Hsu, *Chen's History of Chinese Medical Science*, p. 13.

6. Y. Requena, *Terrains and Pathology in Acupuncture*, p. 43.

7. M. Porkert, *The Theoretical Foundations of Chinese Medicine*, pp. 107–117.

8. Quoted from W. Mann, *Orgone, Reich and Eros*, p. 304.

9. T. Kaptchuk, *The Web That Has No Weaver*, pp. 245–246, 61–62, 232, 228.

10. P. Holmes, "Introduction to Chinese Herbalism" Part Two, *The Journal of Chinese Medicine*, p. 23. From a four part series on Chinese herbalism.

11. L. Fang, "Sun Si Miao," *The Journal of Chinese Medicine*, Vol. 13, p. 4.

12. H. Hsu, op. cit., p. 75.

13. Ibid., p. 99.

Chapter 6

1. G. Vithoulkas, *Homeopathy: Medicine of the New Man*, p. 75.

2. T. Kaptchuk, *The Web That Has No Weaver*, p. 29.

3. H. Roberts, *The Principles and Art of Cure by Homeopathy*, p. 79.

4. J. Kent, *Repertory of the Homeopathic Materia Medica*.

5. J. Kent, *New Remedies, Clincal Cases, Lesser Writings*, pp. 500–501.

6. E. Nash, *Leaders in Homeopathic Therapeutics*, p. 50.

7. K. Mathur, *Principles of Prescribing*, pp. 383–384.

8. Ibid., pp. 3935–397.

9. M. Blate, *The Tao of Health*, p. 39.

10. J. So, *A Complete Course in Chinese Acupuncture*, pp. 15–16.

11. T. Kaptchuk, op. cit., pp. 237–238.

12. Quoted in J. Evans, *Mind, Body and Electromagnetism*, pp. 50–51.

Chapter 7

1. E. Whitmont, *Psyche and Substance: Essays on Homeopathy in the Light of Jungian Psychology*, pp. 54, 130.

2. *U.S. Dispensatory*, 25th Ed., p. 20.

3. D. Bensky, *Chinese Herbal Medicine, Materia Medica*, p. 438.

4. *Essentials of Chinese Medicine*, p. 41.

5. B. Katzung, *Basic and Clinical Pharmacology*, p. 63.

6. M. Porkert, *The Essentials of Chinese Diagnostics*, p. 118.

7. J. Clark, *A Dictionary of Practical Materia Medica*, pp. 931–932.

8. *U.S. Dispensatory*, 25th Ed., pp. 1489–90.

9. J. Kent, Lectures on *Homeopathic Materia Medica*, p. 958.

10. Quoted in *Homeopathic Drug Pictures*, M. Tyler, p. 364.

11. T. Kaptchuk, *Product Guide: Jade Pharmacy*, p. 2:18.

12. D. Bensky, op. cit., p. 646.

13. C. Cheung, *Dialectical Differential Diagnosis and Treatment*, pp. 12, 13.

14. Ibid, pp. 12, 13.

15. *Essentials of Chinese Acupuncture*, p. 69.

16. N. Wiseman, *Fundamentals of Chinese Medicine*, p. 236.

17. C. S. Cheung, op. cit., pp. 11, 12.

18. E. Hamilton, *The Flora Homeopathica*, p. 329.

19. T. Kaptchuk, op. cit., p. 231.

20. J. Clark, op. cit., p. 211.

21. J. Kent, op. cit., p. 620.

22. E. Whitmont, op. cit., p. 132.

23. Lecture notes from Catherine Coulter.

24. C. Cheung, op. cit., p. 12.

25. T. Kaptchuk, op. cit., p. 212.

26. S. Hahnemann, *The Chronic Diseases*, p. 373.

27. Ibid., p. 373.

28. M. Weiner, *The Complete Book of Homeopathy*, p. 150.

29. M. Tyler, *Homeopathic Drug Pictures*, p. 107.

30. Ibid., p. 107.

31. Ibid., p. 107.

32. Quoted in *The Web That Has No Weaver*, p. 54.

33. T. Kaptchuk, op. cit., pp. 45–46.

34. Ibid., p. 46.

35. J. Clark, op. cit., p. 338.

36. From conversations with Dr. Ming Tat Wong (medical doctor and Chinese herbalist).

37. Y. Requena, *Terrains and Pathology in Acupuncture*, pp. 78–79.

38. N. Wiseman, op. cit., pp. 118–125; and G. Maciocia, *Tongue Diagnosis in Chinese Medicine*, pp. 108–109. (see plate #4 for an excellent photograph of this type of tongue.)

39. J. Kirschman (director), *Nutrition Almanac*, p. 86.

40. J. Clark, op. cit., p. 1139.

41. T. Kaptchuk, op. cit., p. 236.

42. Ibid., p. 44.

43. C. Cheung, op. cit., p. 20.

Chapter 8

1. H. Hsu, *Chen's History of Chinese Medical Science*, p. 91.

2. J. Clark, *A Dictionary of Practical Materia Medica*, pp. 321–322.

3. D. Bensky, *Chinese Herbal Medicine: Materia Medica*, p. 656.

4. Ibid., p. 656.

5. There are few reliable books on this interesting subject in the English language. One curious book, which unfortunately does not include much medical diagnosis, is *Secrets of the Face* by Lailang Young, Little, Brown, and Co., 1984.

6. M. Blackie, *The Patient, Not the Cure*, p. 156.

7. Ibid., p. 156.

8. M. Lappé, *When Antibiotics Fail.*

Resources

Homeopathic Books and Tapes

Homeopathic Educational Services
2124 Kittredge Street
Berkeley, CA 94704

National Center for Homeopathy
1500 Massachusetts Ave. NW #41
Washington, DC 20005

Homeopathic Research

Foundation for Homeopathic Education and Research
5916 Chabot Crest
Oakland, CA 94618

Oriental Medical Books

Redwing Books
44 Linden Street
Brookline, MA 02146

Bibliography

Note: Titles marked with an asterisk are particularly recommended.

Bioenergetic Phenomenon:

*Becker, Robert O. *The Body Electric, Electromagnetism and The Foundation of Life.* New York: William Morrow and Company, Inc., 1985.

Boirac, Emile. *Our Hidden Forces: An Experimental Study of the Psychic Sciences.* New York: Frederick A. Stokes Company, 1917.

Brunler, Oscar. *Rays and Radiation Phenomena.* Los Angeles: De Vorss, 1950.

*Burr, Harold Saxton. *Blueprint for Immortality: The Electric Patterns of Life.* London: Neville Spearman, Ltd., 1972.

Coddington, Mary. *In Search of the Healing Energy.* New York: Destiny Books, 1978.

*Evans, John. *Mind, Body and Electromagnetism.* Great Britain: Element Books, Ltd., 1986.

*Grossinger, Richard. *Planet Medicine: From Stone Age Shamanism to Post-Industrial Healing.* Revised edition. Berkeley: North Atlantic Books, 1987.

Krieger, Dolores. *The Therapeutic Touch: How to Use Your Hands to Help or to Heal.* Engelwood Cliffs, New Jersey: Prentice Hall, Inc., 1979.

Krippner, Stanley, and Rubin, Daniel. *The Kirlian Aura: Photographing the Galaxies of Life.* New York: Anchor Press/Doubleday, 1974.

Lakhovsky, Georges. *The Secret of Life: Cosmic Rays and Radiations of Living Beings.* Mokelumne Hill, California: Health Science Press, n.d.

Lowen, Alexander. *Bioenergetics.* New York: Penquin Books, 1975.

*Mann, Edward. *Orgone, Reich and Eros: Wilhelm Reich's Theory of Life Energy.* New York: Simon and Schuster, 1973.

Motoyama, Hiroshi. *Theories of the Chakras: Bridge to Higher Consciousness*. Wheaton, Illinois: The Theosophical Publishing House, 1981.

Reichenbach, Karl von. *The Odic Force: Letters on Od and Magnetism*. London: Hutchinson and Co., 1926.

Russell, Edward Wriothesley. *Report on Radionics: Science of the Future, The Science Which Can Cure Where Orthodox Medicine Fails*. Suffolk, England: Neville Spearman, 1973.

Shepard, Stephen Paul. *Healing Energies: A System of Preventing Disease by Studying the Blueprint of the Body*. Provo, Utah: BiWorld Publishers, 1981.

Thakkur, Chandrashekhar G. *Introduction to Ayurveda: The Science of Life*. New York: ASI Publishers, Inc., 1974.

Westlake, Aubrey T. *The Pattern of Health: A Search for a Greater Understanding of the Life Force in Health and Disease*. Great Britain: Element Books, Ltd., 1985.

Homeopathy:

Allen, H. C. *Keynotes and Characteristics with Comparisons*. Republished. Wellingsborough, England: Thorsons Publisher, Ltd., 1978.

Blackie, Margery G. *The Patient, Not the Cure*. Santa Barbara, California: Woodbridge Press Publishing Company, 1978.

*Boericke, William. *Pocket Manual of Homeopathic Materia Medica*. New Delhi, India: Indian Books and Periodical Syndicate, 1982.

Boger, C. M. *Boenninghausen's Characteristics and Repertory*. Reprint. New Delhi, India: Jain Publishers, 1952.

Boger, C. M. *Studies in the Philosophy of Healing*. Reprint. Bombay, India: Roy and Company, 1952.

Boiron, Jean; Abecassis, Jacky; and Belon, Philippe. *Aspects of Research in Homeopathy: Volume I*. Lyon, France: Boiron, 1983.

Burnett, Compton J. *The Diseases of the Liver: Jaundice, Gall-Stones, Enlargements, Tumours and Cancer: And Their Treatment*. Reprint. New Delhi, India: Jain Publishing Company, 1982.

Clarke, John Henry. *A Clinical Repertory to the Dictionary of Materia Medica.* Essex, England: C. W. Daniel, 1971.

Clarke, John Henry. *A Dictionary of Practical Materia Medica.* Essex, England: C. W. Daniel, 1962.

Cook, Trevor M. *Samuel Hahnemann: The Founder of Homoeopathic Medicine.* Wellingsborough, England: Thorsons Publishers, Ltd., 1981.

*Coulter, Catherine. *Portraits of Homoeopathic Medicines,* Berkeley: North Atlantic Books, 1986.

Coulter, Harris L. *Divided Legacy: The Conflict Between Homoeopathy and The American Medical Association, Volume III.* Berkeley: North Atlantic Books, 1973.

Coulter, Harris L. *Divided Legacy: A History of the Schism in Medical Thought, Volume I and II.* Washington, D.C., Wehawken Book Company, 1977.

*Coulter, Harris L. *Homoeopathic Science and Modern Medicine: The Physics of Healing with Microdoses.* Berkeley: North Atlantic Books, 1981.

*Cummings, Stephen, and Ullman, Dana. *Everybody's Guide to Homeopathic Medicines.* Los Angeles: J. P. Tarcher, Inc., 1984.

*Dhawale, M. L. *Principles and Practice of Homoeopathy, Volume I.* Bombay, India: Karnatak Publishing House, 1967.

Dunham, Carroll. *Lectures on Materia Medica.* Reprint. New Delhi, India: Indian Books and Periodicals Syndicate, n.d.

Farrington, E. A. *Comparative Materia Medica.* New Delhi, India: Indian Books and Periodicals Syndicate, 1982.

Farrington, E. A. *Clinical Materia Medica.* New Delhi, India: Indian Books and Periodicals Syndicate, 1981.

*Gibson, D. M. *First Aid Homoeopathy in Accidents and Ailments.* London: The British Homoeopathic Association, 1982.

Hahnemann, Samuel. *The Chronic Diseases: Their Peculiar Nature and Their Homoeopathic Cure.* Reprint. New Delhi, India: B. Jain Publishing Company, 1981.

Hahnemann, Samuel. *Organon of Medicine.* Republished. Los Angeles: J. P. Tarcher, Inc., 1982.

Hamilton, Edward. *The Flora Homoeopathica*. New Delhi, India: B. Jain Publishers, 1982.

Jouanny, Jacques. *The Essential of Homeopathic Therapeutics*. France: Laboratories Boiron, 1980.

Jouanny, Jacques. *The Essentials of Homeopathic Materia Medica*. France: Laboratories Boiron, 1980.

Julian, O. A. *Materia Medica of New Homoeopathic Remedies*. Beaconsfield, England: Beaconsfield Publishers, Ltd., 1971.

Kent, James Tyler. *Lectures on Homoeopathic Materia Medica*. Reprint. New Delhi, India: Indian Books and Periodicals Syndicate, 1974.

Kent, James Tyler. *New Remedies: Clinical Cases, Lesser Writings, Aphorisms and Precepts*. Reprint. New Delhi, India: B. Jain Publishers, 1981.

Kent, James Tyler. *Repertory of the Homoeopathic Materia Medica*. New Delhi, India: Indian Books and Periodicals Syndicate, 1982.

*Koehler, Gerhard. *The Handbook of Homoeopathy*. Wellingsborough, Enland: Thorsons Publishing Group, 1983.

Lilienthal, Samuel. *Homoeopathic Therapeutics*. Reprint. New Delhi, India: B. Jain Publishing Co., 1983.

Mathur, Kailash Narayan. *Principles of Prescribing: Collected from Clinical Experiences of Pioneers of Homoeopathy*. New Delhi, India: B. Jain Publishers, 1983.

Mathur, Kailash Narayan. *Systematic Materia Medica of Homoeopathic Remedies*. New Delhi, India: B. Jain Publishers, 1979.

Nash, D. B. *Leaders in Homoeopathic Therapeutics*. Reprint. New Delhi, India: Indian Books and Periodicals Syndicate, 1983.

Phatak, S. R. *A Concise Repertory of Homoeopathic Medicines*. Bombay, India: The Homoeopathic Medical Publishers, 1963.

Rawat, P. S. *A Self-Study Course in Homoeopathy*. New Delhi, India: B. Jain Publishers, 1980.

*Roberts, Herbert A. *The Principles and Art of Cure by Homoeopathy*. Essex, England: Health Science Press, 1982.

*Shadman, Alonzo Jay. *Who is Your Doctor and Why?* New Canaan, Connecticut: Keats Publishing, Inc., 1958.

Shaikh, A. M. *Homoeopathy for Colleges.* Belgium: Homoeopathic
   Medical College Publishers, 1974.
*Sharma, C. H. *The International Manual of Homoeopathy and
   Natural Medicine.* Wellingsborough, England: Thorsons Pub-
   lishing Group, 1975.
Shepard, Dorothy. *Homoeopathy for the First-Aider.* Essex, En-
   gland: Health Science Press, 1945.
Smith, Trevor. *A Woman's Guide to Homoeopathic Medicine.*
   Wellingsborough, England: Thorsons Publishers, Inc., 1984.
Tyler, M. L. *Homoeopathic Drug Pictures.* Essex, England: The
   C. W. Daniel Company, Ltd., 1982.
Tyler, M. L. *Pointers to the Common Remedies.* Reprint. New
   Delhi, India: Indian Books and Periodicals Syndicate, n.d.
Weiner, Michael and Goss, Kathleen. *The Complete Book of
   Homeopathy.* New York: Bantam Books, 1987.
*Ullman, Dana. *Homeopathy: Medicine for the 21st Century.*
   Berkeley: North Atlantic Books, 1988.
Ullman, Dana. *Monograph on Homeopathic Research.* Berkeley:
   Homeopathic Educational Services, 1981.
Ullman, Dana. *Monograph on Homeopathic Research, Volume
   II.* Berkeley: Homeopathic Educational Services, 1986.
Vannier, Leon. *Homeopathy: Human Medicine.* London: The
   Homeopathic Publishing Company, Ltd., n.d.
Vithoulkas, George. *Homeopathy: Medicine of the New Man.* New
   York: ARCO Publishing, Inc., 1980.
*Vithoulkas, George. *The Science of Homeopathy.* New York:
   Grove Press, Inc., 1980.
Whitmont, Edward C. *Psyche and Substance.* Berkeley: North
   Atlantic Books, 1980.
*Wright Hubbard, Elizabeth. *A Brief Study Course in Homoeop-
   athy.* St. Louis, Formur, 1977.

Note: Books reprinted in India are difficult to date properly. Many
of these classics are over a hundred years old.

Oriental Medicine, Philosophy and History:

Amsel, Allan. *This is China*. New York: Exeter Books (Simon & Schuster), 1981.

Beijing College of Traditional Chinese Medicine, et al. *Essentials of Chinese Medicine Acupuncture*. Beijing: Foreign Languages Press, 1980.

*Beijing Medical College. *Common Terms of Traditional Chinese Medicine in English*. Beijing: Beijing Medical College, n.d.

Bensky, Dan, and Gamble, Andrew. *Chinese Herbal Medicine, Materia Medica*. Seattle: Eastland Press, 1986.

Blate, Michael. *The Tao of Health*. Davie, Florida: Flakyneor Books, 1978.

Chan, Wing-Tsit. *Chinese Philosophy*. Princeton: Princeton University Press, 1963.

Chang, Stephen Thomas. *The Complete Book of Acupuncture*. Millbrae, California: Celestial Arts, 1976.

Cheung, C. S., and Lai, Yat Ki. *Principles of Dialectical Differential Diagnosis and Treatment of Traditional Chinese Medicine: Current Interpretation*. San Francisco: Traditional Chinese Medical Publisher, 1980.

Chia, Mantak and Maneewan. *Awakening the Healing Energy through the Tao*. New York: Copen Press, 1981.

Connelly, Dianne M. *Traditional Acupuncture: The Law of the Five Elements*. Colombia, Maryland: The Center for Traditional Acupuncture, Inc., 1979.

Djen, Gwei-Lu, and Needam, Joseph. *Celestial Lancets: A History and Rationale of Acupuncture and Moxa*. Cambridge, England: Cambrige University Press, n.d.

Eckerman, Peter. *Closing the Circle*. Fairfax, California: SHEN Foundation, 1983.

*Eisenberg, David, and Wright, Thomas Lee. *Encounters with Qi*. New York: W. W. Norton and Company, Inc., 1985.

Fulder, Stephen. *The Tao of Medicine*. New York: Destiny Books, 1980.

Fung, Yu-Lan. *A Short History of Chinese Philosophy*. New York: The Free Press, 1948.

Heren, Louis, et al. *China's Three Thousand Years: The Story of a Great Civilization.* New York: Collier Books (MacMillan), 1974.

Holbrook, Bruce. *The Stone Monkey.* New York: William Morrow and Company, Inc., 1981.

Hsu, Hong-Yen, and Peacher, William G. *Chen's History of Chinese Medical Science.* Taiwan: Modern Drug Publishers Co., 1977.

Huard, Pierre, and Wong, Ming. *Chinese Medicine.* New York: World University Library (McGraw-Hill Book Company), 1968.

*Kaptchuk, Ted J. *The Web That Has No Weaver: Understanding Chinese Medicine.* New York: Congdon and Weed, 1983.

Lawson-Wood, Denis and Joyce. *Acupuncture Handbook.* Rustington, England: Health Science Press, 1964.

Leslie, Charles. *Asian Medical Systems: A Comparative Study.* Berkeley: University of California Press, 1976.

Li, Dun J. *The Ageless Chinese: A History.* New York: Charles Scribner's Sons, 1978.

Lo, Benjamin. *The Essence of T'ai Chi Ch'uan.* Berkeley: North Atlantic Books, 1979.

Lu, Henry C. *The Chinese Classics of Tongue Diagnosis in Color.* Vancouver, Canada: The Academy of Oriental Heritage, 1980.

Lu, Henry C. *The Yellow Emperor's Classic of Internal Medicine and the Difficult Classic.* Vancouver, Canada: The Academy of Oriental Heritage, 1978.

*Maciocia, Giovanni. *Tongue Diagnosis in Chinese Medicine.* Seattle: Eastland Press, 1987.

*Mann, Felix. *Acupuncture: The Ancient Chinese Art of Healing and How It Works Scientifically.* New York: Vintage Books, 1962.

Mann, Felix. *The Meridians of Acupuncture.* London: William Heinemann Medical Books, Ltd., 1964.

Mann, Felix. *The Treatment of Disease by Acupuncture.* London: William Heinemann Medical Books, Ltd., 1974.

Matsumoto, Kiiko, and Birch, Stephen. *Five Elements and Ten Stems.* Higganum, Connecticut: Paradigm Publications, 1983.

*Needham, Joseph (abridged by Colan Ronan). *The Shorter Science and Civilization in China.* Cambridge, England: Cambridge University Press, 1978.

Needham, Joseph. *The Grand Titration: Science and Society in East and West.* Toronto: University of Toronto Press, 1969.

Ni, Hua-Ching. *The Book of Changes and The Unchanging Truth.* Malibu, California: The Shrine of the Eternal Breath of Tao, 1983.

*Ni, Hua-Ching. *Tao, The Subtle Universal Law and the Integral Way of Life.* Malibu, California: The Shrine of the Eternal Breath of Tao, 1979.

O'Connor, John, and Bensky, Dan. *Acupuncture: A Comprehensive Text.* Chicago: Eastland Press, 1981.

Pomeranz, Bruce, and Stux, Gabriel. *Acupuncture, Textbook and Atlas.* New York: Springer-Verlag, 1987.

Porkert, Manfred. *The Essentials of Chinese Diagnostics.* Zurich: Chinese Medical Publications, Ltd., 1983.

Porkert, Manfred. *The Theoretical Foundations of Chinese Medicine: Systems of Correspondence.* Cambridge, Massachusetts: The MIT Press, 1974.

Requena, Yves. *Terrains and Pathology in Acupuncture: Volume I.* Brookline, Massachusetts: Paradigm Publications, 1986.

Rose-Neil, Sidney. *Acupuncture and the Life Energies.* New York: ASI Publishers, Inc., 1981.

Siu, R. G. H. *Ch'i: A Neo-Taoist Approach to Life.* Cambridge, Massachusetts: The MIT Press, 1974.

Siu, R. G. H. *The Tao of Science: An Essay on Western Knowledge and Eastern Wisdom.* Cambridge, Massachusetts: The MIT Press, 1957.

So, James Tin Yau. *A Complete Course in Chinese Acupuncture.* Watertown, Massachusetts: New England School of Acupuncture, 1977.

So, James Tin Yau. *The Book of Acupuncture Points.* Brookline, Massachusetts: Paradigm Publications, 1985.

Swadesh, Morris. *Conversational Chinese for Beginners.* New York: Dover Publications, Inc., 1948.

Unschuld, Paul U. *Nan-Ching: The Classic of Difficult Issues.* Berkeley: University of California Press, 1986.

Veith, Ilza. *Huang Ti Nei: The Yellow Emperor's Classic of Internal Medicine.* Berkeley: University of California Press, 1949.

Wexu, Mario. *The Ear Gateway to Balancing the Body: A Modern Guide to Ear Acupuncture.* New York: ASI Publishers, Inc., 1975.

Williamson, H. R. *Chinese.* New York: David McKay Co., Inc., 1977.

Wiseman, Nigel, and Ellis, Andrew. *Fundamentals of Chinese Medicine.* Brookline, Massachusetts: Paradigm Publications, 1985.

Worsley, J. R. *Is Acupuncture for You?* Leanington Spa, England and Columbia, Maryland: The College of Traditional Chinese Acupuncture and the Centre for Traditional Acupuncture, 1973.

Science and its New Frontiers:

Benson, Herbert. *The Mind/Body Effect: How Behavioral Medicine Can Show You the Way to Better Health.* New York: Simon and Schuster, 1979.

Bernard, Claude. *An Introduction to the Study of Experimental Medicine.* New York: Dover Publications, Inc., 1957.

Bertalanffy, Ludwig von. *General System Theory: Foundations, Development, Applications.* New York: George Braziller, 1968.

Bohm, David. *Wholeness and the Implicate Order.* London: Ark Paperbacks, 1980.

Capra, Fritjof. *The Turning Point: Science, Society, and the Rising Culture.* New York: Bantam Books, 1982.

*Capra, Fritjof. *The Tao of Physics: An Exploration of the Parallels between Modern Physics and Eastern Mysticism.* New York: Bantam Books, 1975.

Cajori, Florian. *Sir Isaac Newton's Mathematical Principles of Natural Philosophy and His System of the World.* Berkeley: University of California Press, 1934.

Carrel, Alexis. *Man The Unknown.* New York: Halcyon House, 1935.

DeRopp, Robert S. *Creative and Destructive Forces in Modern Science: The New Prometheans.* New York: Delta Publishing, 1972.

Dossey, Larry. *Beyond Illness: Discovering the Experience of Health.* Boston: New Science Library (Shambhala), 1984.

*Dubos, René. *Mirage of Health: Utopias, Progress and Biological Change.* New York: Harper and Row, 1959.

Gillispie, Charles Coulston. *Dictionary of Scientific Biography.* New York: Charles Scribner's Sons, 1971.

Gillispie, Charles Coulston. *Concise Dictionary of Scientific Biography.* New York: Charles Scribner's Sons, 1981.

Greene, Ralph C. *Medical Overkill: Diseases of Medical Progress.* Philadelphia: George F. Stickley Company, 1983.

*Inglis, Brian. *The Diseases of Civilization.* London: Granada Publishing, Ltd., 1981.

Inglis, Brian. *Fringe Medicine.* London: Faber and Faber, 1964.

Katzung, Bertram G. *Basic and Clinical Pharmacology.* Los Altos, California: Lange Medical Publications, 1982.

Kervan, Louis. *Biological Transmutations and Their Applications in Chemistry, Physics, Biology, Ecology, Medicine, Nutrition, Agriculture, and Geology.* New York: Swan House Publishing Company, 1972.

Lehninger, Albert L. *Biochemistry: The Molecular Basis of Cell Structure and Function.* Baltimore: Worth Publishers, Inc., n.d.

*Locke, Steven and Colligan, Douglas. *The Healer Within: The New Medicine of Mind and Body.* New York: The New American Library (Mentor), 1987.

Loye, David. *The Sphinx and the Rainbow: Brain, Mind and Future Vision.* Boulder: New Science Library (Shambhala), 1983.

Murchie, Guy. *The Seven Mysteries of Life: An Exploration in Science and Philosophy.* Boston: Houghton Mifflin Company, 1981.

Ostrander, Sheila, and Schroeder, Lynn. *Psychic Discoveries Behind the Iron Curtain.* New York: Bantam Books, 1970.

Price, Derek J. de Solla. *Science Since Babylon.* New Haven: Yale University Press, 1961.

Selye, Hans. *The Stress of Life.* New York: McGraw-Hill Book Company, 1956.

Schmid, Alfred. *The Marvel of Light: An Excursus.* London: East-West Publications, 1984.

*Sheldrake, Rupert. *A New Science of Life: The Hypothesis of Formative Causation.* Los Angeles: J. P. Tarcher, Inc., 1981.

Talbot, Michael. *Mysticism and the New Physics.* New York: Bantam Books, 1980.

Walker, Kenneth. *The Story of Medicine.* New York: Oxford University Press, 1954.

*Weil, Andrew. *Health and Healing: Understanding Conventional and Alternative Medicine.* Houghton Mifflin Company, Boston, 1983.

Whyte, L. L. *Aspects of Form: A Symposium on Form in Nature and Art.* Bloomington: Indiana University Press, 1966.

Wilber, Ken. *The Holographic Paradigm and Other Paradoxes: Exploring the Leading Edge of Science.* Boulder: Shambhala, 1982.

Wolf, Fred Alan. *Taking the Quantum Leap: The New Physics for Nonscientists.* San Francisco: Harper and Row, 1981.

Miscellaneous:

Cobb, V. *Logic.* New York: Franklin Watts, 1969.

Fetter, Harvey Wickes. *The Eclectic Materia Medica, Pharmacology and Therapeutics.* Portland, Oregon: Eclectic Medical Publications, 1983.

Grieve, M. *A Modern Herbal: The Medicinal, Culinary, Cosmetic and Economic Properties, Cultivation and Folklore of Herbs, Grasses, Fungi, Shrubs and Trees with All Their Modern Scientific Uses.* New York: Dover Publications, Inc., 1971.

Houston, Jean. *The Possible Human: A Course in Extending your Physical, Mental and Creative Abilities.* Los Angeles: J. P. Tarcher, Inc., 1982.

Kueshana, Eklal. *The Ultimate Frontier.* Chicago: The Stelle Group, 1963.

Lappé, Marc. *When Antibiotics Fail: Restoring the Ecology of the Body.* Berkeley: North Atlantic Books, 1986.

Lust, John B. *The Herb Book*. New York: Bantam Books. 1974.

Mills, Simon Y. *The Dictionary of Modern Herbalism: A Comprehensive Guide to Practical Herbal Therapy*. Wellingsborough, England: Thorsons Publishers, Ltd., 1985.

Muramoto, Naboru. *Healing Ourselves*. New York: Avon Books, 1973.

*Tierra, Michael. *The Way of Herbs: Simple Remedies for Health and Healing*. Santa Cruz, California: Unity Press, 1980.

U.S. Dispensatory. 25th and 26th Edition.

Index

Abrams, Albert, 38, 39, 48, 63
Academy at Dijon, 39
Achille's tendon, 231
Aconite, 180, 181, 182
Acupuncture, 2, 16, 47, 52, 55, 61, 92–94, 143, 144, 227, 231, 232, 243
Acute prescribing 151
Adaptive energy,46, 63, 69, 70
Adrenal, 214, 219
Age of Reason, 26
Aggravation, 77
Agricultural: applications, 45; chemistry, 35; crops, 83; U.S. Dept. of Agriculture, 45
AIDS, 22
Alcohol, 217
Alfalfa, 83
Allergy shots, 74
Allopathic, 3,66, 74, 79, 84, 234
Alrutz, J., 39
Alumina, 221
Alzheimer's, 223
Amazon: 237; basin, 204; jungle, 203
American Indians, 242
Amelioration, 77
Analog, 106
Anatomy, 33, 236
Anesthesia, 52
Angelica, 141
Anima, 33, 63
Animal: electricity, 33; magnetism, 33, 63; spirit, 31
Anthracinum, 187
Anthropologist, 59
Antidepressants, 227
Antimuscarine drugs, 184
Anxiety, 240
Arabia, 29
Arabian physicians, 207
Archaeologists, 59
Archetype, 205, 178
Archeus, 30, 63
Aristotle,
Arizona, 193
Armoring, 44
Arsenicum: 187; *Arsenic 7c,* 83
Arthritis, 83
Asking, 171
Asthma, 78
Astronomy, 29
Atomic cloud chamber, 47, 60
Atoms, 80
Atrophine
Aura, 17, 36, 48

Auric energy, 39, 63
Aurum, 207, 208
Avicenna, 207
Avogadro's number, 80
Ayurvedic, 28, 41, 61, 207, 242

Bach flowers, 242
Back pain and acupuncture, 169
Bactericide, topical, 52
Bagnall, Oscar, 36
Balancing, 149
Baptista, 187
Baraduc, Hippolyte, 36
Barefoot doctor, 109
Barety, E., 37, 38, 63
Baryta carbonica: 221, 222; Barium carbonate, 221, 222
Becker, Robert, 10, 16, 52, 53, 54
Bee venom, 74
Belief, reasoned, 59
Belladonna, 66, 183–185, 187, 191
Ben-cao Gang Mu, 137
Ben-cao-ting Ti-Zhu, 137
Bensky, D., 106
Bergson, Henri, 39, 51, 63
Bernard, Claude, 12
Bertalanffy, Ludwig von, 69
Berylius, John, 218
Bi-metallic currents, 34
Biochemical: 7, 59, 65, 70, 75, 81, 87, 245; medicine, 22, 23, 60, 66; model, 9, 13, 20, 21, 23
Bioelectrical energy, 34
Bioenergetic: emanation, 36; forces, 85; medicine, 23, 25, 59, 61, 87, 115; models, 7, 23, 24, 61, 82; patterns, 81; research, 35, 59; system, 71; therapy, 242
Bioenergetics, 34, 48, 60, 65, 244, 245
Bioenergy: 5, 9, 10, 11, 24, 53, 56, 60, 62, 63, 70, 77, 86, 89, 244, 245; summary of basic properties, 62; synonyms for, 63; visual perception of, 60
Biological plasma body, 48
Biologically closed circuits, 54, 63
Biomorphs, 42
Biophysicist, 52
Bioplasma, 63
Black sun, 209
Bladder, 217
Blate, Micheal, 163
Blondot, Rene Prosper, 36, 37, 57, 63
Blood: 119, 121; deficient, 132, 133; hot, 134; stagnant, 134
Blood circulation system, 54
Bloodletting, 181
Bloodpressure, 69
Blueprint for Immortality, 42
Body, 24, 29
Body Electric, The, 16, 54

Body/mind connection, 70, 87, 206, 243
Boerhaave, 191
Boericke's Materia Medica, 155
Bohm, David, 19, 96
Bohr, Neils, 11, 18, 96
Boils, 188, 193
Boirac, Emile, 39, 60, 63
Boiron Laboratories, 83
Bone fractures, 52
Bones, 219
Boorstin, Daniel, 51
Boyd, W.E., 40, 83
Bradycardia, 208
Brain: left, 68, 100, 101, 103; left neurons, 103; right, 68, 100; right neurons, 103; whole, 103
Breathing, 69
Bridgeman, P.W., 86
British Journal of Chemical Pharmacology, 84
British Medical Journal, 40, 186
Brunler, Oscar, 46, 63, 114, 115
Bruno, Giordano, 32, 53
Bufo rana, 235, 236
Building, 149
Bupleurum, 141
Burnett, Dr., 209
Burr, Harold, 10, 14, 15, 42, 43, 63
Bushmaster, 203

Calcarea carbonica, 211–214, 233
Calcium, 211, 212, 221
Callihan, Paul, 87
Calomel, 215
Caloric energy, 5
Cambridge University, 36, 51
Cancer: 21, 22, 52, 86, 220, 244; radiation, 74; War on, 149
Candida albicans, 22
Cannon, William, 68, 69
Capra, Fritjof, 119
Capsicum, 160
Carbuncles, 188
Carrel, Alex, 8
Casetaking: Oriental, 163–165 (see homeopathic)
Cat scan, 233
Catheterization, balloon, 54
Catholic priests, 23, 24
Cayenne, 73
Centessimal "c", 79
Ceramics, 221
Chairman Mao, 109
Chakra, 219
Chaldea, 29
Chapman, Richard, 93
Chargraff, Erwin, 82
Charite, Hospital de la, 36
Charpentier, 37

Chemical pollutants, 83, 89
Chemistry, 12
Chen Hsiu Yuan, 144
Cherry, Dan, 235
Chi: 47, 51, 61, 63; *and blood*, 131; *stuck, obstructed*, 190; *deficent*, 15, 132, 133, 156, 194; *rebellious, stagnant*, 134
Chi Po, 91, 93
Chiang Kai-shek, 109
Children, 238
Chin dynasty, 107
China Wall, 107
Chinese: culture, 107; herbology, 137–144; medicines, 59, 61, 91, 92, 109
Ching Tan An, 165
Chronic prescribing, 151
Chu Hsi, 51
Circle, 86
Clark, John, 211
Cleaves, 37
Clouds, 86
Club moss, 199
Coal tar, 37
Cobb, Vicki, 102
Cobra, 203
Codeine, 35
Cold: 123; Cold turning to heat, 183, 185; induced disorders, 129; invasion, 183; obstruction, 190; stagnation, internal, 190
Collective unconsciousness, 51
College of Scientific Acupuncture, 165
Color, 139
Columbia University, 45
Coma, 184
Combating disease, 149
Comfrey, 235
Common symptoms, 153
Complementary medicine, 245
Computers, 88
Conception vessel, 4, 9, 143
Confucius, 111
Conjunctivitis, 98
Constitutional: remedy, 157; treatment, 151
Conventional medicine, 82
Convulsions, 196, 235
Copenhagen interpretation of quantum physics, 96
Copernican Revolution, 20
Copper, 41
Corneal oppacities, 193
Cornell University, 43
Cortisone, 78
Cosmic rays, 60
Coulter, Harris, 84
Cowardice, 240
Creative Evolution, 39
Crotona, Italy, 29
Cryptodial phenomena, 60
Crystal configuration, 85

Crystal matrix, 85
Cullen's Materia Medica, 72
Cupping, 231
Cybernetics, 59
Cyclotron, 10

Daksha, Prajapati, 28, 63
Damp heat, 134, 217
Dampness: 128, 134, 213, 214; excess, 217; move, 217
Dandelion, 235
Daphne mezerum, 161
Darras, Claude, 95
Davies, Humphrey, 221
De La Warr, George, 45, 60
De Lipinay, 37
De Roches, Colonel, 36
Deadly nightshade, 183, 235
Deductive: 111; logic, 100
Deficient liver blood with wind and deficient kidney yin, 136
Degeneration: 21, 22; Degenerative diseases, 86
Delusions, 183
Dental fillings, 215
Department of Defense, 58
Depression, 240
Descartes, Rene, 24, 31, 32, 58, 114
Devitalized food products, 99
Diabetes, 22
Diacyanine, 36
Diagnosis, 97, 98
Deaphoretic, 191
Diastase, 83
Dielectric biocosmic energy, 46, 63
Dietary practice, 238
Digital, 106
Digitalis, 74, 239
Dilution: 66, 78, 79, 86; centessimal, 79
Direct moxa, 166
Disease: 171, 245; environmentally caused, 46
Disharmony patterns, 25, 171, 179, 227, 245
Disorders: biochemical, 22; emotional/mental, 22
Distension, 206
Diuretic, 191
Divided waters (shui fen), 143
Dizziness, 164, 168
DNA, 6, 13, 82, 103
Dossey, Larry, 19
Driesch, Hans, 30, 40, 43, 51, 53, 63
Drugs: biphasic actions of, 79; pharmacological, 20, 23, recreational, 22
Druids, 201
Drysdale, John, 186
Dualistic concept, 114
Dulcamara, 191, 192
Dunham, Carrol, 161

Dyes, radio opaque, 36

Earaches, 184
Earth, 124, 125, 212
Eastern: 8; model, 26
Eaton, Ralph, 32
Eckman, Peter, 103
Ecology, 11
Eczema, 78
Edema, 213
Eeman, E., 45
Egypt, 29
Eight branches, the, 136, 230
Eight principals, the, 116, 123
Einstein, Albert, 11, 18, 19, 50
Eisenburg, David, 91
Ejection of Energy from Chakras and Meridians, 47
Elan vital, 39, 63
Electric current, 33
Electrical engineer, 61
Electrician, 61
Electro magnetic pollution, 52
Electro-dynamic, 14, 15, 42, 43, 63
Electro-neurophysiology, 34
Electro-static fields, 42, 63
Electro magnetic fields, 23, 42
Electronic devices, 232
Emanometer, 40
Emergency, 141
Emotionals, 153
Emotions: 24, 237
Emperor, 140
Empty, 123
Endocrine glands, 70
Endorphin, 94
Energetic pattern, 76
Entelchy, 40, 51, 63
Entropy, 51, 62
Enzyme, 83, 87
EPI (external pernicious influence), 135
Epidemic, 67
Epilepsy: 235; epileptic, 165
Epstein-Barr virus, 22
Equilibrium, 8
Esoteric knowledge, 26
Eupatorium perfoliatium, 160
Exterior, 123
External cold, 182
External pathogenic factors, 182, 183

Face reading, 236
FDA, 44
Fear, 220, 223
Feedback mechanism, 69
Fertilizers, 83
Fevers: 68; high, 68
Field, nonelectrical, 10
Fields of Life, The, 14, 42

Fight or flight, 214, 219
Fire: 125; deficiency, 214; Fire in the life door (ming men), 166; Fire poison, 188
First aid, 238
Five phases, the: 116, 125, 128; correspondence, 127
Flu, 184
Fludd, Robert, 30, 36, 63
Fluid, The, 63
Fluids: 86, flow, 47
Fog
Folk medicine, 73
Force vitale, la, 36
Forgetfulness, 210
Formative: causation, 51; energy, 63
Foundation for Homeopathic Education and Research, 84
Four elements, 128, 129
Four examinations, the, 116
Four roles, the, 140, 141
Four stages, the, 131, 186
Free siver ions, 52
Frerichs, 38
Freud, Sigmund, 44
Frog-leg experiments, 34
Full: 123; fire, 135; heat, 185
Fungicides, 215, 218

Galileo, 23, 24, 28, 32, 53
Gall bladder, 202
Galvani, Luigi, 33, 34
Gamble, Andy, 106
Gandhi, Mahatma, 65
Gardenia, 141
Gate Theory, 94
Gelsemium, 79
Gem elixir, 207
General symptoms, 153, 157
General Systems Theory, 59, 69
Genetic engineering, 245
Gentian, 41
Gentian dispersing the liver tea, 141
Gestalt: concepts, 149, 172; psychology, 68
Ginseng, 238
Goethe, 178
Gold sodium thiomalate, 208
Gonorrhea, 165
Gravitational, 11
Great Britain, 65
Gregory, James, 35
Gregory, William, 35, 57
Grief, 70, 223
Grieve, M., 180
Grunewald, Fritz, 41
Gun powder, 107
Gurvich, Alexander, 40, 43, 63
Gymnastics, 29

Hahnemann Medical College, 77

Hahnemann, Samuel, 3, 5, 33, 66, 72–75, 78, 178, 179, 208, 221
Hallucinations, 183
Han Dynasty, 107
Harmonic: 73; resonance, 71
Harmony, 29, 149
Harvard: 70; Department of Physics, 86
Harvey, William, 54, 108, 245
Hay fever, 84
Headaches, 164, 184
Healing: 242, 244, 245; response, 68, 70, 71
Health, 8, 68–71, 242, 244
Hearing, 220
Heart, 207–210
Heart, remedy, 208
Heat: 97, 123; excess, 136; Heat of deficient yin affecting the blood, 167
Heisenberg, Werner, 11, 18
Helmholtz, Herman von, 38
Helmont, Jan Baptista von, 30, 63
Hemisync, 103
Hemoglobin, 48
Hepatitis, 98
Herbal energetics, 137–140
Herbalist, Chinese, 137
Herbs: Chinese, 137–140; taste, 139; thermal properties, 139
Hering's Law, 77
Hering, Constantine, 77, 203, 218
Higgins, Eugene, 42
High blood pressure, 22, 98, 164
Higher mind, 100
Hippocrates, 29, 30, 63, 73, 238, 243
Hohenheim, Theophrastus Bombastus von, 30
Holistic: approach, 243; medicine (see medicine), 243; model, 8, 22; pattern, 18; perspective, 24, 242, 243; theory, 243
Holographic: paradigm, 50, 96; theory, 96
Holomotion, 96
Holoverse, 96
Homeopathic: casetaking, 75, 76, 151, 158, 159; following cases, 158, 159; drug response, 75; materia medica, 75; prescribing, 76, 158; scientific research, 82–86
Homeopathic Science and Modern Medicine, 84
Homeopathy: 3, 65–89, 152–163; home and first aid, 238
Homeopathy: Medicine for the 21st Century, 84
Homeostasis, 68, 69, 87
Horder, Lord, 40
Hormesis, 80, 81
Hormones: 80, 81; sex, 80, 81
Horseradish, 218
Houston, Jean, 28, 103
How to Measure and Diagnosis Meridians

and Their Corresponding Organs, 47
Huang Ti, 28, 63, 91, 108
Human atmosphere, the, 36
Human emanations, 46
Humbolt, Alexander von, 34
Huna, 29
Huo To, 108
Huxley, Aldous, 94
Huxley, Thomas, 32
Hydraulics, 107
Hydrolysis, 83
Hygiene, 108
Hyoscamine, 184
Hypertension (see high blood pressure) 22, 98
Hypnosis, father of, 33, 98
Hypnotic phenomena, 33
Hysteria, 210

Iatrogenic, 23
IBM, 49
Ice: 86; crystallization, 86
Ideogram, 105
Ignatia, 160
Immune: deficiency, 22; deficiency diseases, 89; system, 70
Impotent, 203, 220, 221
India, 28, 207
Inductive: 111; reasoning, 102; sciences, 102, 137
Inflammatory process, 69
Insomnia, 164, 165, 168, 228
Institute of Bioenergetic Analysis, 48
Insulin, 67
Interior, 123
Internal wind, 198, 199
International Congress of Experimental Psychology, 39
International Research Institute in India, 51
Intestines, 52, 217
Intonation, 105
Inyushin, Y., 48, 63
Iodine, 106
Irrigational system, 107
Itch, suppressed, 78

James, William, 67
Japanese Acupuncture Association, 47
Jing, deficient, 219–221
Joints, swollen, 173
Jung, Carl, 51, 178
Jupiter, moons of, 24, 28

Kahunas: 29; priests, 29, 100
Kammerer, Paul, 41, 63
Kaptchuck, Ted, 106, 166
Karagrulla, Shafica, 60
Kent's Repertory, 155, 156
Kent, James Tyler, 155, 193, 204

Ki, 47, 63
Kidney: 122, 213, 218, 219, 220; *chi*, 220; *deficient in fire*, 185; *deficiency*, 133, 219, 220, 228; deficient, 220, 228; *fire*, 197, 198; *jing*, deficient, 222, 223; *yang*, 133, 166, 219, 220;*yin*, 133, 223, 228
Kilner, Walter, 36, 63
Kirilian photography, 17, 48
Kirlian, Seymon & Valentina, 17, 48
Koch, R., 21, 239
Korshet, 41
Korshivelt, 46
Krause, 83
Krieger, Dolores, 48
Kritzinger, H.H., 46

L-fields, 42, 63
Lachesis, 178, 203–207, 240
Lamarkian Genetic Theory, 41
Lancet, The, 40, 67, 84, 169
Language, 104
Lao Tzu, 11
Large intestine-11 (wu chi), 186
Laser, 49
Law of similars, 66, 71, 73, 74
Lead, 41
Leaders in Homeopathic Therapeutics, 160
Left brain (see brain)
Lehninger, Albert, 56
Leptons, 18
Less is more, 78
Leyden Jar, 10
Li, 11, 40, 51
Li Shi-zhen, 108, 137
Libido, 205
Licorice, 141
Liebault, Ambroise, 39
Liebig, Justus, 35, 53
Life: 24; energy, 61; fields, 42; force, 34, 63
Like cures like, 66, 73
Linear, 82
Linnaeus, 191
Liquid, 85
Liquid crystals, 49, 86, 87
Listening, 117
Listlessness, 210
Liver: 142, 199, 200, 202; *blood deficiency*, 202, 203; *constriction*, 206; *deficient yang*, 136; *energy invading the stomach*, 176; *fire blazing*, 98; *in excess*, 164, 185; *overheating*, 217; *yang in excess*, 164, 206, 233; *yang rising*, 98, 177, 195, 197, 227
Living energy, 86
Low back pain, 156, 169, 213, 238
Lowen, Alexander, 48
Lower mind, 100
Lu-gen (rhizoma phragmitis communis), 144

Lungs: 10, 213, 144; *deficient blood,* 136; *deficient chi,* 136; *deficient yin,* 135, 136
Luys, Dr., 36
Lycopodium, 199–203, 233, 240
Lyssin, 239

Ma quian zi, 196
Macau Institute of Chinese Medicine, 166
Magic bullets, 149
Magnetic: force, 33; radiation, 39
Magnetics, 49
Magnetism, animal, 33, 38
Malaise, 208
Malaria, 72
Mammals, 52
Manning, Clark, 148, 168
Margenau, Henry, 42
Margrou, Madame, 43
Marx, Groucho, 169
Masturbation, 235
Materia medica, 155, 156
Mathematics, 18, 29
Matter and Memory, 39
Maxwell, J.C., 37
McCarthy era, 44
Mechanism: 58; model, 95; thought, 59, 82, 96
Meddygon Myddofai, 180
Meditation, 17, 234
Medicine: 29; bioenergetic, 25, 33, 60; Chinese, 3, 4; holistic, 2, 25; Oriental, 226; testing of bioenergetic, 60
Memory, poor, 210
Mendel, Gregor, 41
Mentals, 152
Menstrual flow, 207
Mercurachrome, 215
Mercurius: 215; *chloride,* 83
Mercury, 215
Meridian system: 120, 121; of acupuncture, 98, 120, 121; Chinese organ system, 121, 122; twelve, 166
Mesmer, Franz Anton, 33, 63
Messenger herbs, 140, 141, 142
Metabolism, 214, 219
Metal phase, 125
Metallurgy, 47
Mezerum, 161
Microdoses, 65–87
Microscope, 10, 95
Microwaves, 52
Middle ear, 214
Middle warmer, 191, 228
Migraines, 77
Miller, Robert, 47, 60, 63
Millikan, Prof., 60
Millman, S., 45
Mind, 24, 29
Minister herbs, 140–142

Mister Sulphur, 179
Mitogenetic radiation, 43, 63
Modalities, 154, 172, 237
Modern drugs, 20
Monkshood *(aconite)* 180–183, 235
Monroe Institute, The, 103
Monroe, Robert, 103
Morphine, 35
Morphogenic fields, 12, 13, 15, 51, 63
Moss, Thelma, 17, 49
Motion sickness, 75
Motoyama, Hiroshi, 47, 63
Moxabustion, 144, 191, 228, 231, 238
Mucus, 134
Muller, Erich, 41, 42
Murex purpurea, 159, 160
Music, 29
Mustard gas, 84

N-rays, 37, 63
Nadis, 41
Nancy, France, 37
Narcotics, 191
Nash, E.B., 160
Natural law, 59, 88
Naturalists/Chinese, 137
Nature, 32
Nausea, 183, 208
Needam, Joseph, 5, 92
Needle biopsy: 15; percutaneous, 54
Nei Ching (Inner Classic), The, 28, 73, 91
Nerve energy, 38
Nerve radioactivity, 39, 63
Nervous system, 70
Neuric energy, 38, 63
New Concepts in Diagnosis and Treatment, 38
New Science of Life, A, 13, 51, 58
Newton, Isaac, 18, 24, 31, 32, 50, 96, 102
Newton-Cartesean: model, 27, 31; Newtonian, 21; Newtonian model, 18
Night urine, 168, 169
Nightshades, 191
Nitric Acid, 207
Nitroglycerine, 74, 239
Nonconducters, 41
Nordenstrom, Bjorn, 10, 15, 54, 55, 61, 63
Northrup, F., 42
Nosodes, 186, 230, 239
Nuclear, 11
Nuclear magnetic resonance spectroscopy, 81
Nurturing, 149
Nux vomica, 176, 178, 195–199, 206, 227, 233

Objectives, 155
Odic force, The, 34, 35, 47, 63
Opium, 35

Optics, 49
Organ systems, 70
Organ transplants, 245
Organon of Medicine, The, 33, 73
Orgone: 44, 47; accumulators, 44; energy, 63
Oriental Medical Doctors (OMD), 115, 165
Osteopathy, 242
Our Hidden Forces, 39, 60
Overcooling, 185
Overheating, 185, 187, 188
Oyster, 211, 235

Paeonia lactiflora, 168
Painkillers, prototypic, 184
Palestine-Phoenicia, 29
Palpation, 117
Palpitations, 210
Paracelsus, 3, 30, 63, 73, 178
Paradigms, 8
Paraelectricity, 47, 63
Parafin, 34
Parasympathetic nervous system, 184
Particular symptoms, 153, 157
Pasteur Institute, Paris, 43, 239
Pasteur, Louis, 21
Pathology, 20
Pathos, 66
Patterns: 111; of disharmony, 25, 97, 115, 119, 149, 227; semi-crystalline, 86
Patterson, 89
Peculiar symptoms, 153, 154, 157
Pediatric care, 108
Penicillin, 67, 188, 240
Pennsylvania Farm Bureau Co-Operative, 45
Peoples Republic, The, 107
Persia, 29
Personality, 210
Pets, 238
Philodendrum leaf, 49
Philosophy, 18, 29
Phosphorus, 157
Photoelectric, 218
Physical energy, 38, 39, 63
Physical symptoms, 153, 156
Physics: 9, 12; modern physicists, 115
Physiology, 51, 236
Physis, 30, 63
Pictogram, 103
Pien Chueh, 116
Pierrakos, John, 48, 49
Placebo: 81, 89; response, 67
Plank, Max, 27
Plant research, 49
Plato, 13, 178
Pneuma, 10, 29, 63
Pneumonia, 165
Poison nut, 195

Polarity Therapy, 242
Polychrest remedies, 196, 211
Polygonum multiflorum, 168, 223
Polymers, high, 47
Polypharmacy, 13
Pomeranz, Bruce, 93
Porkert, Manfred, 121
Possible Human, The, 28, 103
Potency: 80, 81; Potentizied, 79, 80; Potentizing, 86
Prague University, 46
Prana, 10, 20, 47, 49, 63
Prat, Sylvester, 44
Premature aging, 220
Preventive medicine, 98
Principia Mathematica, The, 31
Proving: 73, 74, 75; crude, 75
Psychic energy, 39, 63
Psycho energetic fields, 63
Psycho-energetics, 50
Pulmonary lesions, 20
Pulsatilla (windflower), 76, 163, 179
Pulse: irregular, 210; Pulse-taking, 117, 118
Pyrogen, 186–188
Pythagoras of Samos, 29, 58, 63

Quantum: physics, 17, 18, 47, 67, 96; packets, 237; theory, 96
Quarks, 18
Quartz crystal, 49
Quasi electrostatic fields, 63
Queen Elizabeth II, 65
Quinine, 72, 160
Quintessence, 30, 63

Rabi, I.I., 45
Radar, 52
Radiation: devitalizing, 41; vitalizing, 41
Radio: 52; transmitter, 45
Radioactive: isotope, 95, tracer, 83
Radiology, 15
Radionics, 38, 40, 42, 44, 45, 242
Rahn, Otto, 43
Ramus, 32
Rattlesnake, 203
Ravitz, Leonard, 15, 42, 43
Rayonnante Et Circulante, Le, 21
Rays and Radiation, 46
Regeneration: 16, 22, 40, 52, 62; rats limb, 52; power, 20
Rehmannia glutinosa, 141, 168, 223
Reich, Wilhelm, 10, 43, 44, 48, 58, 63
Reichenbach, Karl von, 10, 34, 35, 63
Reichian Therapy, 242
Remedies: 66; pictures, 149; types, 233
Renaissance, 28, 58, 59, 67
Repeating, 141, 142
Report on Radionics, 38
Reproduction, 40

Requena, Yves, 119, 131
Resonance, 77, 149
Restlessness, 210
Restructures, 86
Rheumatoid arthritis, 84, 168, 169, 208
Rhus toxicodendron, 173, 231
Richards, Guyon, 42, 63
Ries, Stanley, 83
Roberts, Herbert, 151
Rockefeller, John D., 67
Rockwell, B.A., 45
Rosicrucian order, 32
Royal family, 65
Royal Society of Medicine, 40
Ruta, 231

Sage, 235
Salamander, 53
Salty flavors, 220
Sanderson, Burden, 108
Sanscrit, 242, 244
Scarlet fever, 184
Schizophrenia, 15
Schlemmer, Jan, 44
Science, 81, *Science*, 83
Scutellaria, 141
Seasons, 237
Sedation, 238
Seizures, 165
Selenium, 218–221, 239
Selye, Hans, 46, 47, 63, 69
Semantics, 106
Semiconductor, 218
Senile, 223
Sensations: 154, 155; as if . . . 154
Sepia, 159, 160, 179
Seven recipes, the 141, 142
Sex hormones (see hormones), 214
Sexual: disfunctions, 213; symptoms, 155
Shang-Hun Lun (Discussion of Cold Induced Disorders), 129, 183
Shao yang, 130
Shao yin, 130, 183
Sheldrake, Rupert, 13, 30, 40, 51–52, 63
Shen, 206–208, 210
Shen-Nung, 137
Shi gao (gypsum, calcium sulfate), 144
Shock, 240
Shui fen (cv-9), 143
Signs, 236
Simba, 238
Simillar disease, 73
Simillimum, 76, 155, 156
Six energetic layers (see six stages)
Six interactions, 140, 141
Six stages, 116, 129–130, 183
Skin disease, 191
Sleep, 155
Sleeping pills, 227

Slippery, 118, 214, 228
Slow, 118
Smelling, 117
Snow, 85
Societe de L'Harmonie Universalle, 33
Socrates, 13
Solanaceous alkaloids, 183, 184
Sore throat, 184
Soul, 29
Spirit, 210
Spleen: 212#214, 238, -9, 143; Damp, 226; deficient, 228
Stahl, George, 32, 33, 63
Stanford University, 50
Stannum, 193–195, 221
Stephenson, 81
Stoerck, Anton von, 180
Stomach: 212, 228, 239; -36, 144; -43, 144
Stress, 68, 69, 99
Stroke, 236
Strontium, 221
Structured, 86
Strychnine, 196
Stubborness, 214
Su Wen, 210
Subatomic: particles, 18; world, 18, 19
Subtle flame, 31
Subtle spirit, 31
Succussion: 66, 79, 86; succussed, 79
Sugar, 240
Sulphur, 179, 211, 218, 231, 235
Sulphuric acid, 207, 218
Summer heat, 235, 236
Sun Su Mo, 144
Suspension bridge, 107
Swann, 239
Sympathetic vibration, 71
Syncope, 208
Synthesis, 231
Syphilis: 215; syphlitic miasm, 216
Systemic lupus erythematosus, 167
Systems Theory of biology, 68
Syzygy, 112
Szent-Gyorgyi, Albert, 129

Tachon, 60
Tai chi, 234, 238
Tai yang: 130, 183; disturbances, 136
Tai yin, 130
Tan Chi Chu, 108
Tao: 9, 112–114; Taoism, 107; Taoist, 99; monad, 112, 96; philosophy, 113
Tao Hong-jing, 137
Tao of Health, The, 163
Tao of Physics, The, 19
Tapeworms, 193
Tarentela, 187
Teeth, 220
Temper, 206

Temperature control, 69
Template, 81
Terrains and Pathology in Acupuncture, 131
Tesla, Nikolai, 17
Theraputic Touch, The, 48
Thermodynamics, 62
Three yellow calming the spirit tea, 141
Thyroid gland, 108, 214, 219
Tibetan medicine, 242
Tiller, William, 50, 65,
Time and Free Will
Tin, 193
Tiny doses, 73
Tissue regeneration, 52, 53
Tobacco, 75
Tokyo University, 47
Tongue, 116, 118, 217
Tonification, 238
Touching, 117, 118
Toxic: side effects, 78, 87; toxicity, 73; toxicological reports, 175
Trace elements, 218
Transliteration, 103
Trauma, 135, 240
Trialistic, 114
Triple warmer, 213
Tsan Tien Chi, 165
Tubercullinum, 186, 239
Tumors, 16
Twain, Mark, 67

Ulcers, 191
Ullman, Dana, 84
Ultimate Frontier, The, 59
Unified: bioelectric force field, 6, 9; Energy System, 97
Unifying force, 244
Unitary force, 243
University of: Bolagna, 33; Edinburgh, 35; Geissen, 35; Jena, 40; Montreal, 46; Munich, 35; Nancy, 37; Tubingen, 34; Upsala, 54; Vienna, 43; Yale, 42, 43
Upton, Curtis, 45

VA hospital, Syracuse, 52
Vaccines, 74
Vanrenen, Louis, 148, 221
Vegetable sulfur, 199
Veterinarian application, 45
Vibration de la Vitalite Humaine, Les, 36
Virchow, 38
Vis medicatrix naturae, 30, 63
Vital energy, 12
Vital force, 5, 33, 51, 63
Vitalism, 12, 27, 43, 47
Vitalistic: 34; research, 37
Vitamins: 232; vitamin E, 218
Vogel, Marcel, 49
Voll, Rheinhold, 232

Volta, Alessandro, 34, 57
Vomiting, 183

War on Cancer (see cancer)
Warts, 191
Washington, George, 215
Wasserman, 38
Water: 86, 87; molecules, 85
Watson, James, 102, 103
Weak-interacting, 11
Weather: 46, 237; artificial conditions, 46
Wei, 131
Weir, John F., 197
Weiss, Paul, 13, 51
Western: 24; civilization, 240; diet, 240; medicine, 59; model, 8
Westlake, Aubrey, 44, 45
Wheeler, 19
Whitmont, Edward, 178, 179
Whyte, L.L., 171
Will, 29
Wind, 31, 97, 198
Wind invading the surface meridians obstructing the Chi and Blood, 167
Wiry, 118
Wisdom of the Body, The, 68, 69
Wise Judge, 195
Wolfsbane, 180
Wood, 124–129, 202
Wood disharmony invading stomach and intestines
Wood, Robert, 37, 58
Woody nightshade, 191
Worrall, Ambrose, 47
Worralls (unit of measurement), 47

X-rays, 37, 60, 81, 221, 233
Xylonite, 44

Yang: 8, 9, 19, 112–115, 116, 119, 120, 135; deficient, 131–136, 167, 168
Yin ling quan (Yin hill spring), 143
Ying, 131, 186
Yoga, 238

Zang fu, 222
Zhang Zhong-jing, 108, 129, 137, 183
Zhi-zhi (Fructus gardeniae jasminoides), 144
Ziegler, 41, 46

About the Authors

Clark Manning, raised in Oklahoma, was headed for a career in biology when he discovered Chinese medicine. He then began a long and multifaceted education in the healing arts, a path that included acupuncture, herbalism, flower essences, and nutritional medicine, as well as homeopathy. After graduation from the New England School of Acupuncture, he and Louis engaged in a detailed study of homeopathy which gradually evolved into this book. Among his many teachers, Clark studied with Marcel Vogel, research scientist and crystal expert. Clark, a cross-country skiing enthusiast who also appreciates classical music, belongs to the New England Sound Healers Association, and practices T'ai Chi. For the past seven years he has worked in partnership with Louis Vanrenen in a clinic south of Boston.

Louis Vanrenen, born in Zimbabwe (Rhodesia) of English parents, has had a lifelong interest in foreign cultures and medicines. He has had the good fortune to travel extensively in Asia, Europe, Mexico, and Africa, gaining first-hand experience of traditional medicines and different cultures. Louis graduated from the University of Colorado where for six years he studied "everything," his special interests being poetry and biology. After graduation from the New England School of Acupuncture, he worked with a variety of acupuncturists, medical doctors, and homeopathic physicians. Presently Louis practices acupuncture and homeopathy, studies such diverse fields as biochemistry, shamanism and radiesthesia, and lives in Marshfield, MA., with Johnna Albi and their two children, Gabriel and Ariana, with whom he enjoys trekking in mountains and deserts.